BMA

The Changing Face of Volunteering in Hospice and Palliative Care

D1375698

The Changing Face of Volunteering in Hospice and Palliative Care
An international perspective

Edited by

Ros Scott
Honorary Research Fellow, University of Dundee,
UK and Co-chair, EAPC Task Force on Volunteering
in Hospice and Palliative Care

Steven Howlett
Deputy Director, Roehampton University Business School,
London, UK

OXFORD
UNIVERSITY PRESS

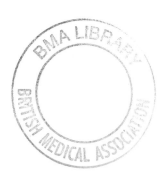

OXFORD

UNIVERSITY PRESS

Great Clarendon Street, Oxford, OX2 6DP,
United Kingdom

Oxford University Press is a department of the University of Oxford.
It furthers the University's objective of excellence in research, scholarship,
and education by publishing worldwide. Oxford is a registered trade mark of
Oxford University Press in the UK and in certain other countries

First Edition published in 2018

Impression: 1

Published in the United States of America by Oxford University Press
198 Madison Avenue, New York, NY 10016, United States of America

British Library Cataloguing in Publication Data

Data available

Library of Congress Control Number: 2017959064

ISBN 978–0–19–878827–0

Printed in Great Britain by
Ashford Colour Press Ltd, Gosport, Hampshire

Foreword

The discipline of palliative care is primarily focusing on the patient who has the disease—whether it be cancer or other chronic diseases. It is crucial to take psychosocial issues into consideration in order to deliver optimal palliative care. The patient-centered approach ought to be combined with a disease-centered approach in order to deliver optimal care. This combined approach is expected from the patients, the family and from society.

Most textbooks in medicine focus mainly on the disease approach. This approach is well covered, including new knowledge about the pathology, the epidemiology, the diagnosis and the treatments of the disease. However, knowledge and competence in psychosocial issues are needed in order to combine the disease and patient centered approach; this combination is seen in "early integration of palliative care."

Already, in 2002, the World Health Organization (WHO) changed some of the content of their definition of palliative care. It clearly states some fundamental issues related to organization, content and competence in palliative care:

+ For patients and families "facing the problems associated with life threatening illness"

+ From an organizational perspective: "palliative care is applicable early in the course of illness, in conjunction with other therapies that are intended to prolong life"

+ It should be performed "through the prevention and relief of suffering by means of early identification and impeccable assessment and treatment"

+ It constitutes a broad approach to the patients "assessment and treatment of pain and other problems, physical, psychosocial and spiritual"

Four main issues are debated today with background in the content of the WHO definition. These issues are also relevant for the need of psychosocial care:

Integration of palliative care early in the disease trajectory

+ A correct use of diagnostic tools , and methods to identify patients in need of treatment

+ Family involvement – a life threatening disease will also have impact on the family

+ Patients with life threatening diseases are often suffering from several symptoms and signs in parallel of physical, psychosocial and spiritual nature

Psychosocial issues in palliative care is content wise one of the main pillars of modern palliative care.

This book covers main areas of psychological and social care and the important role of volunteers. Many of the chapters give excellent updates, and more than that; the book is discussing fundamental approaches to patient care and health care. The need for a community-based approach involving volunteers is necessary in order to reach a basic goal in palliative care to give the patients the possibility to stay at home as much and for as long as possible, and to die at home if desired. The latter goals will probably need to be facilitated by involving end of life care in community care as well as a part of the national public health policies. This book is therefore highly relevant for clinicians in general and even more for palliative care specialists and all those who work in palliative care.

Contents

Contributors List

Stephen Claxton-Oldfield
Associate Professor, Department of Psychology, Mount Allison University, Canada

Anne Goossensen
Professor of End of Life Volunteering, University of Humanistic Studies, Utrecht, The Netherlands

Nigel Hartley
Chief Executive Officer, Earl Mountbatten Hospice, Isle of Wight, UK

Michaela Hesse
Department of Palliative Medicine, University Hospital Bonn, Germany

Steven Howlett
Deputy Director, Roehampton University Business School, London, UK

Alex Huntir
Palliative Care New South Wales, Australia

Fatia Kiyange
Programmes Director, African Palliative Care Association, Kampala, Uganda.

Piotr Krakowiak
Head of Department of Social Work, Nicolaus Copernicus University, Toruń, Poland

Sara Morris
Senior Research Associate, International Observatory on End of Life Care, Lancaster University, UK

Anil Kumar Paleri
Consultant, Palliative Medicine and Clinical Director, Palliative Care Society, Kozhikode, Kerala, India

Leszek Pawłowski
Department of Palliative Medicine, Medical University of Gdańsk, Poland

Sheila Payne
Emeritus Professor, International Observatory on End of Life Care, Lancaster University, UK

Leena Pelttari
CEO Hospice Austria and Co-chair of the EAPC Task Force on Volunteering in Hospice and Palliative Care, Austria

Anna H. Pissarek
PR and Project Coordination, Hospice Austria, Austria

Lukas Radbruch
Department of Palliative Medicine, University Hospital Bonn and Malteser Hospital Seliger Gerhard Bonn Rhein-Sieg, Germany

Heather Richardson
Joint Chief Executive, St
Christopher's Hospice and
Honorary Professor, Lancaster
University, UK

Libby Sallnow
Palliative Medicine Registrar,
University College London Hospital,
and Doctoral Student, University of
Edinburgh, UK

Greg Schneider
Founder and President, Hospice
Volunteer Association, USA

Ros Scott
Honorary Research Fellow,
University of Dundee, UK and
Co-chair, EAPC Task Force on
Volunteering in Hospice and
Palliative Care

Jos Somsen
Formely Policy Advisor at VPTZ
Nederland and Independent Health
Care Policy Advisor, The Netherlands

List of Abbreviations

AHD	Ambulante Hospizdienste		Bundesinstitut für Gesundheitswesen
AIDS	acquired immunodeficiency syndrome	GP	general practitioner
ART	antiretroviral therapy	HEAL	Hospice Educators Affirming Life
ASHA	Accredited Social Health Activists	HIPAA	Health Insurance Portability and Accountability Act
AVSM	Association of Voluntary Service Managers	HIT	Health Information Technology
BAME	black and minority ethnic groups	HITECH Act	Health Information Technology for Economic and Clinical Health Act
CAF	Charities Aid Foundation	HIV	human immunodeficiency virus
CBVs	community-based volunteers		
CBWs	community-based workers	HPC	Hospice and palliative care
CCWs	community care workers	HPCO	Hospice Palliative Care Ontario
CHA	Under the Canada Health Act	HPG	hospice and palliative care law
CHBC	community home based care	HR	human resources
CHPCA	Canadian Hospice Palliative Care Association	IiV	Investing in Volunteers
CHWs	community health workers	IPM	Institute of Palliative Medicine
CMS	Centers for Medicare and Medicaid Services	Khanya-aicdd	Khanya—African Institute for Community Driven Development
CoPs	Conditions of Participation	LSGI	Local Self Government Institutions
CPCA	Canadian Palliative Care Association (Later changed to CHPCA see above)	LTC	long-term care
CS	Caritas Socialis	MCCM	Medicare Care Choices Model
DOT	Directly Observed Therapy	NCD	non-communicable diseases
EAPC	European Association for Palliative Care	NCVO	National Council for Voluntary Organisations
ECEPT	Eastern and Central European Palliative Care Task Force	NGO	non-government organisation
EHR	Electronic Health Record	NHS	National Health Service
EU	European Union	NNPC	Neighbourhood Network in Palliative Care
FLSA	Federal Fair Labor Standards Act	NPOs	non-profit organizations
German DRG	Diagnosis Related Groups	NSW	New South Wales
GÖG/ÖBIG	GÖG/ÖBIG Gesundheit Österreich GmbH / Österreichisches	OAMGMAMR	Order of Nurses Midwives and Medical Assistants in Romania

ONS	Office for National Statistics	VNAs	Visiting Nurses Associations
OVC	other vulnerable children	VPTZ	Volunteers in Palliative Care The Netherlands
PaTz	Palliative Care in the Home situation	VTZ	Volunteers Terminal Care foundation
PC	palliative care		
PDV	Patient Data Vault	WPCA	Worldwide Palliative Care Alliance
PHC	primary health care	WHA	World Health Assembly
PLHIV	people living with human immunodeficiency virus	WHAT	Hospice Voluntary Work as a Tool of Acceptance and Tolerance for People Leaving Penal Institutions
RVH	Royal Victoria Hospital		
SIPC	Students in Palliative Care	WHO	World Health Organization
SOM	Services State Operations Manual	WIIFM	What's In It For Me?
SAVP	specialized palliative home care	WLRCT	wait-list randomised controlled trial
TB	tuberculosis		
UNV	United Nations Volunteers		

Chapter 1

The modern context of volunteering

Steven Howlett

Introduction

The idea for this book came when the editors produced the second edition of *Volunteers in hospice and palliative care: A resource for voluntary services managers* (Scott et al., 2009). That volume contained practitioner-written chapters on *how* to manage volunteers, offering a 'state of the art' view of good practice, but the volume also included an additional chapter on how volunteering for palliative care was organized in Kerala. The chapter gave a counterpoint perspective to organizing and involving communities in palliative care different from almost everything else in the book. Readers and reviewers picked up on this chapter praising how it piqued their interest to think about volunteering and palliative care in new and different ways. It was also evident that even since that book, a lot has changed in volunteering. Given the fast pace of change and interest volunteer-involving organizations have in encouraging community level—and led—participation, could a Kerala-like model show the way? Would that be possible within existing 'ways of working'? We felt it was a good idea to review how palliative care involved volunteers and reflect on the changes that are happening from the perspective of practitioners and academics in different countries.

But of course it is too simple to believe that any model can be translated wholesale from one country to another. Volunteering is a product of different historical developments and cultural tradition—for example, a reading of Davis Smith's tracking of voluntary action in the UK, takes the reader through the traditions of philanthropy and self-help covering the *noblesse oblige* 'duty to the poor' model while at the same time examining the bottom up self-help history of mutual aid essential to understand why voluntary action looks as it does in the UK today (Davis Smith, 1995). Salamon and Anheier (1998) broadened our understanding when they developed the social origins theory to explain how the prevailing attitudes of ruling classes to welfare expenditure give a particular pattern of voluntary action. Their thinking helps explain why the United Kingdom (UK) is different from Asia and Asia from the Americas and so on. Rolling this forward, Colin Rochester (2013) used the UK to offer a well-crafted critique of how the distinctive nature of voluntary action has been captured and shaped by policy makers. In other words context matters, and if we are to learn new ways of working we need to consider why and how a particular approach works.

It is in this spirit that this book gathers accounts of volunteer involvement in hospice and palliative care across a range of countries and regions. As editors, we asked the contributing authors to tell us about volunteering in hospice and palliative care in their own country. We wanted, of course, some similarity in structure; we asked for a history of volunteering in hospice and palliative care—clearly these had to be snapshots. We asked for developments—what are the changes and trends, and importantly we asked the contributors (a mix of practitioners and academics) what they thought were the facilitators and barriers that were driving those trends. We wanted to be able to see how good ideas were sustained and to be helped to see if those ideas are transferable. In reading the accounts sent to us—we were struck but similarities and differences. The final chapter of this book looks to draw out what we saw as interesting themes. In asking the authors for their accounts we decided not to harmonize language unduly so where you notice differences in terms for volunteers, or community, or for people at the end of life, we ask you to read with that in mind. In some cases the authors tell us exactly why a term is chosen; in other cases it is up to us to reflect on how language results from context and tradition and how it may, in itself, influence current and future practice. The only rule we set was for the book to talk about 'involving' volunteers and avoid 'using' volunteers; though the reader will note that in Greg Schneider's chapter the *Conditions of Participation* from the Department of Health and Human Services does just that.

This first chapter gives an overview of the modern context of volunteering by looking at trends and research about volunteering in general to offer a context for the chapters that follow. So much has been written about volunteering and its reach can be seen almost anywhere. For example, ask what seems like a basic question: 'what motivates people to volunteer?', (a key concern for all the authors in this volume) and you will soon find more studies than you could comfortably read and assimilate without it becoming a major study. To get a working knowledge a good start would be classic studies by Clary et al. (1992, 1996, 1998) outlining the Functions Index which aims to identify the psychological needs that motivate volunteers and, in turn, should help volunteer managers attract and keep volunteers by fulfilling those needs. After that it really depends on what specialized area is of interest— for example the role altruism plays in decisions to volunteer (see Burns et al., 2006)—or the social and political context that motivates students to volunteer. For example, see Hustinx et al. (2010) for a study comparing motivations across six countries. Young people, after all, will be the volunteers of the future and because we see that in the UK the trend in declining number of hours given to regular volunteering is reversed in the 16–24-year-old age group, according to the Office for National Statistics (ONS, 2017a) we may want to know more about how to engage the young. Or maybe your organization still sees older volunteers as your key source of volunteers. If so, then start with Okun et al., (1998) to tease out the different motives for older volunteers. We could go on. If you are asking 'what about hospice and palliative care volunteers?', you need only search for the works of Stephen Claxton-Oldfield whose account of volunteering in Canada appears in this volume. And yet, for all the studies, one report in the UK quoted a practicing volunteer manager as commenting: 'Motivation is one of the most over-researched topics [but] none of the research really gives a practitioner anything valuable because everyone's different' (quoted in Saxton et al., 2015: 35).

As people with a keen interest and some involvement in researching volunteering we would argue that this perhaps goes too far and that there is much value in the insights research brings to all aspects of volunteering, not least motivation. But we also note that the ever closer examination by volunteering researchers into narrower and narrower specialities, in ever expanding sectors, and into different organizations maybe leaves those readers frustrated who want a more holistic view. This is, in turn, not to overlook the work of organizations and publications that specifically look to present readable, practice-focussed work—such as the already quoted. (NFP Synergy Reports, the work of organizations like the Institute for Volunteering Research in the UK or e-volunteerism in the United States). These, and others, present research-based ideas for discussion in such a way that practitioners and academics can engage with each other. To those we hope to add this book. It can be read as accounts and stories (indeed readers will see how powerfully volunteers tell their own stories in Chapter 15 and in the stories of Compassionate Neighbour volunteers in Chapter 14 by Sallnow and Richardson). In the final chapter (Chapter 16) we summarize some of the points that are worthy of comparing and contrasting when thinking in terms of community development as much as volunteer management development, about the pros and cons of national structures for standards and just how important is it that there is some government-led policy backdrop acknowledging the work of volunteers?

The rest of this chapter offers a necessarily short background look at what we know about the people who volunteer, about the organizations they participate in, and how governments are shaping the volunteering environment. It draws on UK data to show what trends are seemingly emerging and it errs towards volunteering in general to hopefully set questions in mind for the reader for the subsequent chapters.

People who volunteer

Knowing how many people volunteer always presents some difficulties because figures derived from surveys depend on how the survey was constructed and conducted; we know that how a question on volunteering is phrased can dramatically alter the response (Lyons et al., 1998). Comparisons over time *within* countries often need explanations and caveats to take account of different questions asked and different survey methodologies and attempts at international comparisons merely magnify the challenges (Rochester et al., 2012). At the time of writing up to date figures appeared in the Charities Aid Foundation (CAF) World Giving Index for 2016. This covers both the giving of time and money. The challenge of interpreting figures is clear immediately because the report gives figures for 'helping a stranger' and 'volunteering time'. We may argue that the former is part of the latter. Even taking the latter as a formal action performed through an organization the global league table makes us pause; Turkmenistan has top position which it had held from 2011 until the 2015. The reason given for its slipping from top spot in 2015 was that 'Saturday Subbotnik's' had been cancelled. Subbotniks were times when people were 'expected' to volunteer during the Soviet era (Davis Smith, 2001 references Subbotniks in his review of the relationship between volunteering, the state, and democracy). That is to say, there is a question about how voluntary the volunteering was. The country's return to the top of the rankings may show that there is a spirit of volunteering separate from the 'coercive' nature of Subbotniks. It certainly shows that measuring volunteering is not easy. Nevertheless, the CAF report makes some general comments on global volunteering that do help to set a broad picture. It notes that since 2014 there has been a small increase in the proportion of people volunteering their time—from 21.0–21.6 per cent, and that this is an increase from the 2011 benchmark which was 18.7 per cent (CAF, 2016).

Separating out data for the UK in the report shows that 33 per cent of respondents saying they volunteer time, and, as changes over the previous year were only noted where it was a rise or fall of more than three percentage points, we may conclude that the rate of volunteering in the UK remained broadly steady. Figures from the UK Government Community Life survey (noted by the Institute for Volunteering Research as the best source of data) for 2015–16 indicated that 41 per cent of respondents in England volunteered formally at least once in the previous year. It also noted that 27 per cent were 'regular volunteers', that is they said took part at least once a month. Crucially, the figures show no significant changes, which were 42 per cent for all volunteers and 27 per cent for regular volunteers (Cabinet Office, 2016).

The point here is that though the totals may be different from the CAF analysis, *the trend* is the same, broadly speaking the same number of people participate. This is echoed in a study of a number of volunteering surveys in the UK by Staetsky and Mohan (2011). While this may be disappointing for policy makers wanting to encourage more active participation in community life, it does suggest that roughly the same number of people are there and ready to help. A steady number of people volunteering must be good news. But, despite what the volunteer manager quoted above noted, there are developing trends within active volunteers that managers should look to research to explain. These trends will probably alter from place to place and similarities and differences will be evident as the authors of the other chapters describe from their own experience of working with volunteers in hospice and palliative care in different countries. Volunteering data collection, however, is variable. Canada, the US, and the UK have traditions of national surveys of volunteering. When it comes to identifying volunteering in hospice and palliative care it is much harder. While a number of countries collect national hospice and palliative care volunteering data on a regular basis, (see Austria, Chapter 4) at this point in time the UK does not. Some, therefore, may not have national figures to frame their understanding of their own work, but it is noticeable that there is only fleeting worry that palliative care struggles to find volunteers. Scott (Chapter 3) makes the point that despite changes in volunteering in hospices and palliative care services in the UK, by and large attracting volunteers is not problematic. Most of the accounts given in this work have authors identifying fairly stable 'types' of volunteers in terms of age and gender; Claxton-Oldfield notes a 'typical' volunteer as female, white, middle-aged (Chapter 8), or older and not in paid employment or retired. It is the exceptions to this that are notable; for example Palleri and Sallnow specifically note the younger age profile of volunteers within one neighbourhood scheme in India compared to those in other parts of the country (Chapter 12).

Taking this 'steady-state' of volunteering as the backdrop, can we discern trends within it? Using the example of the UK and looking across several sources in the UK we can see, again, a reasonably consistent picture. There is no discernable gender difference between men and women for formal volunteering, but with differences in what each do; women are more likely to provide caring and men representation roles (National Council for Voluntary Organisations (NCVO), 2017). By age group the highest rates of regular volunteering (at least once a month) are in the age groups 16–25 and 65–74 years, the lowest is in the 25–34 years range (NCVO, 2017), figures from the following year show this age difference as even more pronounced. The Office of National Statistics, reporting on time spent volunteering in the UK, finds that between 2012 and 2015 volunteers gave 7 per cent less time to communities over the period, and, when a notional wage is given to this it equates to a 'loss' of more than £1 billion. This research shows that—in line with these figures—the 16–24 year group (note the slightly different grouping) increased the time they gave while for the 25–34 year group time given fell (ONS, 2017a). Analysis by time given also shows that although participation rates between sexes is the same, women gave an average 1.50 hours a week in 2015 while for men it was 1.19 hours. The picture seems mixed, but again the message is 'broadly stable'. What this chapter does is only to give an illustrative picture for the UK of formal volunteering (through an organization), but the chapters of this book invite comparison of what trends look like and mean in the context of hospice and palliative care volunteering in each country.

The research shows, therefore, that overall volunteer numbers are holding up. Does research indicate that these volunteers are participating for different reasons? We have noted that there is a wealth of research on motivations and a practitioner's more sceptical view of how that research helps. Certainly within the following chapters motivation is a key theme. The volunteers in Sallnow and Richardson (Chapter 14) talk of having a chance to exercise compassion and deepen feelings of community belonging; themes echoed in the volunteer stories in Chapter 15. Kiyange (Chapter 11) in an overview of palliative care across many African countries also noted themes of compassion built out of cultural traditions of community care. But other motivations are evident too— of how volunteering can lead to paid work, and how in areas of poverty payment of a stipend encouraged involvement. While these varying motivations could underline the previous comment that motivations are very individual and so studies can tell us little, we can also reflect and echo more broadly, understanding changing volunteer motivations.

Motivations can be considered from a psychological perspective or a sociological one. The former asks what needs someone is looking to satisfy through volunteering, the latter looks at how people contextualize their involvement (Rochester et al., 2012). The work of Clary and colleagues (1992, 1996, 1998) is framed in psychological thinking with motivation translated as the need to, for example express values, or acquire experience, or to feel that one is giving something back to the community. It has proved to be a compelling model and research often follows the idea of categorizing volunteer 'need' and matching it to volunteer task (for example, see research in event volunteering by Treuren,

2013). Hustinx and colleagues (2010) theorize the sociological perspective in their work on reflexive volunteering in young people. They argue that volunteering is seen as a self-project where volunteering is part of a person's identity. The work of the Pathways to Participation project in the UK can be seen in this light. The volunteers interviewed tell their story, what volunteering means to them, and how it is part of their life (Ellis Paine, 2015). Conclusions drawn from the interviews include that 'There is a need to move beyond explanations of why people volunteer that focus on asking their motivations, and of how people volunteer that focus on isolated volunteering activities' (2015: 1). Chapter 15 of volunteer stories in this volume can be read with this in mind. We can draw out motivations but we can also see how the stories reflect what volunteering means to the volunteer. Perhaps this suggests that the modern context of volunteering is one in which the practitioner needs to be able to synthesize both these views, by looking more holistically at motivations. Studies like 'Pathways to Participation' become as important as volunteer surveys and it as well to be careful that we do not assume survey results carry more weight. One survey listed 10 motivations and asked volunteer managers 'Do you think any of these have become more important to volunteers over the last five years?'. Eighty-one per cent of managers list 'Improving their CVs' as what they saw as an increased motivation to volunteer which 72 per cent identifying 'Developing new skill' and 53 per cent 'Developing existing skills' (Saxton et al., 2015). In fourth place was 'Giving some back' identified by 33 per cent. Religious belief was identified by just two percent even though other surveys indicate that being actively religious has a significant influence on the propensity to volunteer (Low et al., 2007). Perhaps because the survey captured perceptions it may be that these more skills-development motivations are increasing whereas the others remain important but are just not *seen* as becoming more important. Nevertheless, this does seems to resonate with the idea that motivations to volunteer are being driven by more instrumental reasons and that if organizations are to recruit more people their message needs to be broadcast on the What's In It For Me (WIIFM). Underlining this is the idea that '[T]here is little doubt that the current age of austerity, together with more long-standing changes in access to higher education and the competitiveness and composition of the job market, has pushed the salience of employability to the fore' (Saxton et al., 2015: 38).

Motivations then may vary, but what we see here is a weaving of the twin ideas of volunteering being part of a person's identity and for volunteering to offer the volunteer something they can use in other facets of their life. The two are not at all mutually exclusive and how we develop and support volunteering needs an understanding of how these two aspects combine. Back in 1996 Davis Smith noted Peter Drucker's assessment of volunteers transition from well-meaning amateur to a trained, professional member of staff who would expect responsibility, a part in decision making, opportunities to advance, and lots of training (Davis Smith, 1996). Such a model could clearly help volunteers who are looking for experience and transferable skills. It can also help volunteers feel that their time is being well used and appreciated. And yet, there is also a warning that the 'paid work without pay' model can too easily slip into volunteering being managed in such as way it can be less appealing (Rochester, 2013).

Organizations involving volunteers

Having considered who volunteers, we now turn to how volunteers are supported and managed. Much of the research on volunteer motivation emphasizes that the practical application is that by identifying what volunteers want, organizations that meet those motivational needs can expect to have satisfied volunteers. But the task of managing volunteers has more to it than that. Indeed when Drucker suggested that volunteers are trained, professional members of staff (albeit unpaid) there is an implication that the management of those volunteers is equally professional and organized. Volunteers need skilled managers and there continues to be a call that volunteer management should be a profession in itself in the UK (Howlett, 2010; Payne and Morris, Chapter 2). It is not an unreasonable call once the breadth of skills needed to manage an unpaid workforce is appreciated. The chapters in this volume on volunteering in hospice and palliative care give a clear signal of the place of the volunteer manager in successful volunteering; Huntir is in no doubt that the success of palliative care volunteering in Australia is underpinned by organizational support for volunteers, by the skills of volunteer managers and by the inclusion of volunteers in aspects of service management. If Drucker is right and 'training, training and more training' is crucial (Quoted in Davis Smith, 1996: 192) then our contributors have a wealth of knowledge to share.

However, research and writings on managing volunteers urges caution. Rochester et al. (2012) reviewed research on the formalization of volunteering arguing that volunteer management was increasingly adopting the techniques of private and public sector management and that this need not be accepted as an inevitable norm. The theme was taken up by Saxton et al. (2015) in their review of volunteering and volunteer management. They argued that volunteering was being held back by an over acceptance of volunteering as analogous to HR management. Quoting practicing managers they argued that 'fixing systems and processes' was assuming more importance than dealing with people. Even so the authors argue that the HR model

'[I]s not without valuable lessons: supervision and support; the need to consult and set objective; proper legal oversight to protect both parties.' (Saxton et al., 2015: 74).

The argument for well thought out management is a strong one. The idea that volunteers are not passive recipients of tasks given to them by organizations needing 'an extra pair of hands' is not new; back in 1996 Davis Smith noted that there was already a growing sense that volunteers were 'voluntary not amateur', and that they needed supportive and professional management to not only fulfil their tasks for the organization but also because they wanted a meaningful role that could be seen to be making a difference. In this sense volunteering is amenable to and in need of 'management'. Indeed while researching the challenges of volunteer management in health care in the United States of Anerica, Rogers et al. (2013) go on to extent the idea that volunteering should not only be part of an Human Resources (HR) function, but a 'strategic' HR function to better align volunteering to organizational needs and that performance indicators for volunteering needed to be developed. Their argument for management is compelling (what is the best way to ensure your new volunteer doesn't come back for a second day? Tell them to 'sit in the corner and have a cup of tea while we think of something for you to do') but Davis Smith (1996) was also keen to point out that the advance of 'the managerialists' was being resisted, not least by those who saw 'the workplace' model as damaging to that other concept that needs scare quotes—'the spirit of volunteering'. That debate, as we have noted, has been fleshed out and argued thoroughly by Colin Rochester arguing that conceptualizing, and organizing volunteering, as if it is an economic activity—paid work without the pay—may not always be helpful (Rochester, 2013; Rochester et al., 2012). For sure, studies tell us that volunteers want development, skills, to know what they need to do when, and to know where it is possible to use their own initiative. But at the same time we should not ignore that the 'management' school of voluntary action is counter-poised by the organic participatory role (Zimmeck, 2001). By concentrating on training, organization, management, and so forth our authors may simply be in the thrall of the management school. And yet, many are talking about how the 'service' the volunteers provide is being extended out of 'buildings' (hospices and hospitals) and into homes and the community, and explicitly drawing on community development models to grow these activities (for example, see especially Goossensen and Somsen, Chapter 5; Sallnow and Richardson, Chapter 14, in this volume). If we are to consider the modern context of volunteering we need to ensure we are not entirely trapped by notions derived from management thinking. Brudney and Meijs (2014) approach the issue by arguing that where volunteering replicates paid work an HR analogous model is logical, but where the volunteer role is less defined (their research was on volunteers in social work), managers need to be more fluid in their approach.

The debate may seem easier at the extremes—a volunteer giving complex legal advice for example may need regular updating for, de-briefing on cases, supervision on performance, and so on: while volunteers in a hobby club—which is more like Rochester's notion of volunteering as a convivial activity—may need a minimum of organization. But the middle ground is trickier. Read the stories of the volunteers in this volume and you may see people who just want to help and not be subject to a management control, but in the chapters you will also read of roles where specialism is key and management support needed. All of the chapters in this volume have easily identifiable management models and structures and readers will note just how formal some of them are. In other places there are spaces evident for volunteer-led services, initiative, and voice. We asked contributors to identify what works for their contexts and perhaps it is evident that managerial discourse rolls on. And yet, in places—very evidently in the volunteer stories—we still see the importance of that elusive 'spirit of volunteering'.

The policy-makers

We cannot consider the modern context of volunteering without looking at how some of the issues already noted are driven by influences outside volunteer-involving organizations. We often think of volunteering as part of the third sector, and that by implication is not part of the state or market. We would be wrong of course not to think wider than that—much volunteering happens in the public sector. If we take the UK again as an example, volunteers acting within school governance roles number somewhere about 300,000. Although methods of calculating the value of volunteering vary, the Office for National Statistics in the UK put the figure at £22.6 bn, or approximately 1.2 per cent of GDP (ONS, 2017b). Given that scale of contribution it is little surprise that policy makers are keen to encourage more participation. But it is not only the economic contribution which attracts attention, the social benefits of participation are also hugely attractive. Haß and Serrano-Verlade (2015) note that several European countries have instigated national volunteer service programmes largely because alongside the economic argument '[V]olunteering develops forms of civic engagement and solidarity that are vital to the integration of modern societies' (p. 1720). For Ellis Paine and Hill (2016) the benefit is threefold—the distinctive contribution of volunteers, the democratizing of services, and the cost effectiveness. For policy makers volunteering offers a win-win—encouraging participation helps to fix broken parts of society and offers a huge resource.

In the UK we can see the interest and influence of government directly on volunteering. Government programmes start most obviously in the 1970s with the Good Neighbour Campaign (Davis Smith, 1998), since then there have been numerous others. Young people have been catered for by the Millennium Volunteers programme under Labour followed by the Conservative government version of a National Citizen Service. There have at various times been programmes focussed on older volunteers and to encourage employee volunteering. So, on the one hand government have been encouraging volunteering, it seems, because it is the right thing to do. Any of the government-sponsored programmes can fit nicely into wider aims to characterize what a participatory society is. More recently, this took the form of former Conservative Leader and Prime Minister David Cameron's idea of 'The Big Society'. On relinquishing the Prime Ministership to Theresa May, the notion converted into the idea of the 'Shared Society'. Though in truth any of these concepts lack a core idea that is easily understood. Little wonder then that too often the ideas lose traction and volunteering is cast more in its economic possibility than its participatory one. Sir Stuart Etherington, Chief Executive of the NCVO writing on the year ahead for the voluntary sector in January 2017 noted 'It was saddening to see the former prime minister's theme of a big society lost momentum and became derided as simply a cover for cuts' (Etherington, 2017: 3). And there lies a problem: government wants to encourage volunteering, and even puts in place programmes for it, but the lure of a 'free resource' means volunteering is often seen as cover for ever more needs that government struggles to meet. Again reading through the contributions to this book and you may be struck by how many hospice and palliative care services are expanding to meet new demands which are often age related, for example dementia. You may also be struck by how the funding for this comes through one government department or another. Reading the United Nations Volunteers (UNV) *State of the Worlds Volunteerism Report* you will be left in no doubt of the power of volunteering to shape governance (UNV, 2015: xiv) and reading the chapters in this book you will see how hospice and palliative care volunteering too is centred around participation and activism. But it is also clearly about service and how to manage those services.

The context of volunteering for government is how to harness volunteer energy, and that too is about priorities. The future of the National Citizen Service mentioned has recently been questioned by the parliamentary committee that scrutinizes public expenditure as too expensive (BBC, 2017). And yet we know that one of the key indicators of likelihood to volunteer is having done it before (Musick and Wilson, 2008). In other words we know that encouraging young people to be involved in voluntary activity is likely to mean more will be volunteers in the future; we can effectively look forward to future savings (the economic model) and participation will help with citizen education. And yet, the cost now may be too great. The modern context of volunteering could be that we are not looking far enough into the future.

Payne and Morris in Chapter 2 note that the World Health Assembly in 2014 issued a resolution to integrate palliative care into national health care systems. The chapters in this book make reference to the history of hospice and palliative care from, in most cases, its voluntary roots. And while that will probably remain, drawing care into national health systems will most likely have the subsequent effect of increasing rules and procedures to respond to oversight by statutory organizations. Again not necessarily a bad thing, and in many cases it may bring additional funding. The likelihood is however, that this will increase formalization which Payne and Morris note. In such circumstances the criticism mentioned earlier that managers look to systems and overlook people seems an inevitable result of hospice and palliative care being drawn into national health care systems. Of course it need not be inevitable that it happens without sensitivity and oversight. We will see in some of the following chapters that volunteering in hospices and palliative care and the participation of volunteers still has themes of activism of doing something because it is needed irrespective of whether governments are addressing problems. It retains notions of developing services where there is need as well as within institutions of care and it still draws on the willingness of people to work without pay to give something back to the communities in which they live.

References

BBC (2017) *National Citizen Service: Call for 'radical thinking' for voluntary scheme.* Available from: http://bbc.co.uk/news/uk-39260166 [Accessed 14.03.2017.]

Brudney, J.L. and Meijs, L.C.P.M. (2014) Models of volunteer management:Professional volunteer program management in social work. *Human Service Organizations: Management, Leadership and Governance* 38: 297–309.

Burns, D.J., Reid, J.S., Toncar. M., Fawcett, J. and Anderson, C. (2006) Motivations to volunteer: The role of altruism. *International Review on Public and Nonprofit Marketing* 3(2): 79–91.

Cabinet Office (2016) *Research and analysis Community Life Survey 2015 to 2016: data.* Available from: https://www.gov.uk/government/uploads/system/uploads/attachment_data/file/539105/2015_16_community_life_survey_data.csv/preview [Accessed 20.01.2017.]

Charities Aid Foundation (2016) *CAF World giving index 2016.* Availble from: https://www.cafonline.org/about-us/publications/2016-publications/caf-world-giving-index-2016 [Accessed 14.03.2017.]

Clary, E., Snyder, M., and Ridge, R. (1992) Volunteers' motivations: A functional strategy for the recruitment, placement and retention of volunteers. *Nonprofit Management and Leadership* 2(4): 333–50.

Clary, E., Snyder, M., Ridge, R., Copeland, J., Stukas, A., Haugen, J., and Miene, P. (1998) Understanding and assessing the motivation of volunteers: A functionalist approach. *Journal of Personality and Social Psychology* **74**(6): 1516–30.

Clary, E., Snyder, M., Ridge, R., Copeland, J., Stukas, A. (1996) Volunteers' motivations: Findings from a national survey. *Nonprofit and Voluntary Sector Quarterly* **25**(4): 484–505.

Davis Smith, J. (1995) 'The voluntary tradition: philanthropy and self-help in Britain 1500-1945'. In Davis Smith. J, Rochester, C., and Hedley, R. (eds) *An Introduction to the Voluntary Sector*. London: Routledge.

Davis Smith., J. (1996) 'Should volunteers be managed?' In Billis, D. and Harris, M. (eds) V*oluntary Agencies. Challenges of Organisation and Management*. Basingstoke: Macmillan.

Davis Smith, J. (1998) Making a difference: Can governments influence volunteering?. *Voluntary Action* **1**(1) Winter: 7–31.

Davis Smith, J. (2001) 'The Inflatable Log': Volunteering, the State and Democracy'. *Voluntary Action* **3**(3): 13–27.

Ellis Paine, A. (2015) *Telling Tales of Volunteering: Organisational Insights*. A research findings briefing paper. University of Birmingham: Third Sector Research Centre.

Ellis Paine, A. and Hill, M. (2016) The engagement of volunteers in third sector organisations delivering public services. In Rees, J. and Mullins, D. (eds) *The Third Sector Delivering Public Services*. Bristol: Policy Press.

Etherington, S. (2017) *Stuart Etherington's New Year Letter to the Sector*. Available from: https://blogs.ncvo.org.uk/2017/01/16/stuart-etheringtons-new-year-letter-to-the-sector/ [Accessed 16.01.2017.]

Haβ, R. and Serrano-Verlade, K. (2015) When doing good becomes a state affair: Voluntary service in Germany. *Voluntas* **26**(5): 1718–38.

Howlett, S. (2010) Developing volunteer management as a profession. *Voluntary Sector Review* **1**(30): 355–60.

Hustinx, L., Handy, F., Cnaan, R.A., Brudney, J.L., Pessi, A.B., and Yamauchi, N. (2010) Social and cultural origins of motivations to volunteer. A comparison of university students in six countries. *International Sociology* **25**(3): 349–82.

Low, N., Butt, S., Ellis Paine, A. and Davis Smith, J. (2007) *Helping Out: A national survey of volunteering and charitable giving*. London: Cabinet Office.

Lyons, M., Wijkstorm, P. and Clary, G. (1998) 'Comparative studies of volunteering: What is being studied'. *Voluntary Action* **1**(1): 45–54, reprinted in Davis Smith, J. and Locke, M. (eds) (2007) *Volunteering and the test of time*. London: Institute for Volunteering Research.

Musick, M. and Wilson, J. (2008) *Volunteers. A social Profile*. Bloomington and Indianapolis: Indiana University Press.

NCVO (2017) *UK Civil Society Almanac 2017 / Volunteer Profiles*. Available from: https://data.ncvo.org.uk/a/almanac17/volunteer-profiles-4/ [Accessed 02.06.2017].

Okun, M., Barr, A., and Herzog, A.R. (1998) Motivation to volunteer by older adults: A test of competing measurement models. *Psychology and Aging* **13**(4): 608–21.

ONS (2017a) *Billion pound loss in volunteering effort*. Available from: http://visual.ons.gov.uk/billion-pound-loss-in-volunteering-effort-in-the-last-3-years/ [Accessed 17.03.2017.]

ONS (2017b) *Changes in the value and division of unpaid volunteering in the UK: 2000 to 2015*. Available from: https://www.ons.gov.uk/economy/nationalaccounts/ satelliteaccounts/articles/changesinthevalueanddivisionofunpaidcareworkintheuk/ 2015#valuation-of-unpaid-formal-volunteering [Acccessed 25.03.2017.]

Rochester, C., Eliis Paine, A., and Howlett, S. (2012) *Volunteering and society in the 21st century*. Basingstoke: Palgrave Macmillan.

Rochester, C. (2013) *Rediscovering Voluntary Action. The Beat of a Different Drum*. Basingstoke: Palgrave Mcmillan.

Salamon, L. and Anheier, H. (1998) Social origins of civil society. Explaining the non-profit sector cross-nationally. *Voluntas* **93**(3): 213–47.

Saxton, J., Harrison, T. and Guild, M. (2015) *The New Alchemy. How volunteering turns donations of time and talent into human gold*. Available from: https://nfpsynergy.net/ free-report/new-alchemy [Accessed 10.03.2017].

Rogers, S.E. Rogers, C.M., and Boyd, K.D. (2013) *Strategic human resource management of volunteers and the link to hospital patient satisfaction* [Electronic version]. Available from: http://scholarship.sha.cornell.edu/articles/809 [Accessed 31.05.17, from Cornell University, School of Hotel.]

Scott, R., Howlett, S., and Doyle, D. (eds) (2009) *Volunteers in hospice and palliative care A resource for voluntary service managers*, 2nd edition. Oxford: Oxford University Press.

Staetsky, L. and Mohan, J. (2011) *Individual Participation in the United Kingdom: an overview of survey information*. University of Birmingham: Third Sector Research Centre.

Treuren, G.J.M. (2013) Enthusiasts, conscripts or instrumentalists? The motivation profile of event volunteers. *Managing Leisure* **19**(1): 51–70.

UNV (2015) *2015 State of the World's Volunteerism Report. Transforming Governance*. Bonn: United Nations Volunteers.

Zimmeck, M. (2001) *The Right Stuff: New ways of thinking about managing volunteers*. London: Institute for Volunteering Research.

Chapter 2

The modern context
of palliative care

Sheila Payne and Sara Morris

Introduction to contemporary hospice
and palliative care

This chapter focuses on providing a brief introduction to hospice and palliative care from an international point of view. This introduction will first provide some insights into what palliative care and hospice care is, and how quality of palliative care might be assessed. In order to create a better understanding of the role of volunteers within these organizations, we explain more about the diversity in the organizational structures and delivery of palliative care from many parts of the globe. This provides the context for subsequent chapters presenting evidence of volunteering from specific countries and regions. This introductory chapter highlights some of the current public health debates and challenges facing health care systems and governments in which palliative care offers a response to care. The chapter ends by providing a short description of a few studies investigating the role of volunteers drawn from the United Kingdom to illustrate the types of innovative ways that volunteers can be involved in supporting patients and their families as they face advanced disease and the final phase of life.

Caring for dying people and those with advanced and incurable conditions has been a concern for many societies throughout history, but has largely been undertaken within the context of the family. Over the centuries, philanthropic organizations, religious institutions, hospitals, nursing homes, and refuges for the poor and dispossessed have also provided accommodation for the chronically ill and dying. While compassionate care may have been provided in some of these places, most did not combine all aspects of medical care with diligent attention to psychosocial and spiritual needs (Humphreys, 2001). The first modern hospice, St Christopher's Hospice, was opened in 1967 in South London by Dame Cicely Saunders with the aim of offering excellence in clinical care, education, and research, and focusing on the needs of dying patients and their families (Clark, 2002). Since then, the philosophy and practice of palliative care, initially described as hospice or terminal care, has spread worldwide (Payne and Lynch, 2015).

Definition of palliative care

Palliative care refers to enhancing the physical, psychological, emotional, social, spiritual, and existential well-being of patients and their families (Sepulveda et al., 2002). The World Health Organisation (WHO) adopted the following definition of palliative care (Sepulveda et al., 2002: 94):

> Palliative care is an approach that improves the quality of life of patients and their families facing the problems associated with life-threatening illness, through the prevention and relief of suffering by means of early identification and impeccable assessment and treatment of pain and other problems, physical, psychosocial and spiritual.

Palliative care:

- Provides relief from pain and other distressing symptoms
- Affirms life and regards dying as a normal process
- Intends neither to hasten nor postpone death
- Integrates the psychological and spiritual aspects of patient care
- Offers a support system to help patients live as actively as possible until death
- Offers a support system to help the family cope during the patient's illness and in their own bereavement
- Uses a team approach to address the needs of patients and their families, including bereavement counselling, if indicated
- Will enhance quality of life, and may also positively influence the course of illness
- Is applicable early in the course of illness, in conjunction with other therapies that are intended to prolong life, such as chemotherapy or radiation therapy, and includes those investigations needed to better understand and manage distressing clinical complications

A multidisciplinary and holistic approach forms the core of palliative care practice, while allowing for considerable diversity in the implementation of services, their organizational location, and funding across the world. Ideally services should be available to all patients in need of palliative care wherever they are: in hospitals, at home, nursing homes, prisons, and other institutions. Therefore, palliative care should not be limited to a specific setting. Palliative care is suitable across the life span and for patients with any advanced or life-limiting condition. The provision of support for family members throughout the illness trajectory and during bereavement is a core component of palliative care. In some countries there is recognition of different levels of palliative care:

◆ *General palliative care* which is provided by the health care professionals normally involved in the treatment of the patient and family with low- to moderate-complexity of palliative care need, who have a good basic knowledge of palliative care, and

◆ *Specialist palliative care services* which are provided for patients and their families with moderate- to high-complexity of palliative care need and delivered by health care professionals who have additional training and expertise within palliative care

Recommended definitions of common terms used in palliative care have been offered by the European Association for Palliative Care (EAPC) (Payne and Radbruch, 2009, 2010). However, terminology in palliative care is somewhat controversial and varies across, and even within, countries. The terminology used is influenced by the historical development and the nature of health care systems in different countries and changes over time. For example, in the United Kingdom, terminology relating to palliative care has undergone a number of transitions from hospice care and terminal care in the early period of hospice development (1960s and 1970s), to palliative care towards the turn of the last century (1980–2000), and since 2008, end of life care has emerged as the preferred term.

In most but not all countries, volunteers are a key component in delivering palliative care, managing services, and/or obtaining the funds to establish and run services. Palliative care offers opportunities for clinicians and health care workers in other disciplines to work in partnership with volunteers to forge innovative alliances to shape the compassionate care of people facing the final stages of life.

Role of volunteers within hospices

Modern palliative care volunteer roles vary considerably by organization, by country, by health care system, and over time. Different models of delivery, which have grown up in relation to the context and culture of that society, are evident globally (Morris et al., 2013). The settings in which volunteer roles are performed include both community settings, such as the patient's home, and institutional settings, including purpose built hospices, hospital wards, and nursing homes (Woitha et al., 2015). The range of roles which volunteers undertake is wide, from fund raising, to practical tasks, to befriending. Smeding and Mason (2012) identify three groups of volunteering roles which attract different types of volunteer. The first of these are the roles where professionally acquired skills are used, such as in administrative, clinical, and governance positions. Secondly, community-based volunteers who fund raise or provide practical help, such as shopping, gardening, and driving. Then there are the patient and family supportive roles; such as befriending, bereavement support, respite care, or work in hospices that support the notion of 'normality' and connection to everyday life (Morris et al., 2015).

The definition of volunteer roles, however, is often underdeveloped and in practice confusion of 'role boundaries' can occur (Payne, 2001; Low et al., 2005; McKee et al., 2007; Berry and Planalp, 2008; Weeks et al., 2008; Savery and Egbert, 2010; Sevigny et al., 2010). The performance of overlapping roles, such as friend, advocate, and/or go-between, can raise 'boundary' issues that need careful management (Morris et al., 2015). Field-Richards and Arthur (2012) highlight the need for role clarity and transparency in the negotiation of boundaries between paid and unpaid staff. A further aspect of the volunteer role is in community engagement (Scott, 2015). This role is often assumed rather than explicitly defined, contains elements of education, and the potential for community feedback into strategic planning and service delivery. In addition, hospice volunteers can contribute to social bonds that foster a more humane and cohesive community around terminally ill patients (Sevigny et al., 2010). Future-looking policies frequently mention the need to address the roles, identity, and confidence of volunteers. The EAPC Task Force on Volunteers has prepared a charter on volunteering in Hospice and Palliative Care in Europe to highlight the considerable role played by volunteers within this sector (see http://www.eapcnet.eu/Themes/Resources/VolunteeringCharter.aspx).

Why and how hospice and palliative care are changing

Globally approximately 56 million people die each year, with the majority (68 per cent in 2012) dying with, or from non-communicable diseases (NCD), often in older age (World Health Organisation, 2016). The population of Europe, North America, Australasia, and parts of Asia is ageing; increasingly older people live with chronic and advanced conditions before they die. In other parts of the world, such as sub-Saharan Africa, communicable diseases, including HIV/AIDS, tuberculosis, and malaria, place heavy demands on palliative care services. Arguably during the early development of palliative care, there was a strong focus on the effective management of physical symptoms, especially pain relief, in patients with advanced cancer (Clark, 2002). This has erroneously led to an assumption that palliative care is only appropriate for those with cancer. The section 'Population needs for palliative care' examines the question of who needs palliative care, and what are the pressures upon the sector in responding to contemporary public health challenges.

Population needs for palliative care

The world's population is ageing with the number of people over 60 years expected to double from about 11 per cent to 22 per cent between 2000 and 2050. Most people will die in late old age following a slow dying trajectory with multiple comorbidities, some degree of sensory or cognitive disability, and often complex palliative care needs (Van den Block et al., 2015). The four main NCDs include cardiovascular disease, cancer, diabetes, and chronic lung diseases, with three quarters of all NCD deaths in 2012 occurring in low- and middle-income countries, as cited by the WHO (2016). According to Cancer Research UK, there were 8.2 million cancer deaths worldwide, with over half of all deaths occurring in low- and middle-income countries. The WHO have estimated that the number of people living with dementia worldwide will double to 65.7 million by 2030 and triple to 115.4 million by 2050 (Hall et al., 2011). A recent analysis has estimated that in high-income countries 69–82 per cent of dying people would benefit from access to palliative care (Murtagh et al., 2014). It has been estimated that globally 20 million people with advanced disease need palliative care in the last year of life, and a further 20 million people need end of life care annually, as reported by the WHO and Worldwide Palliative Care Alliance (WHO and WPCA, 2014).

There are great disparities in the availability of palliative care across the world (The Lien Foundation, 2015). Globally, the majority of patients who are diagnosed with cancer have advanced disease which is no longer amenable to curative treatment. This means that they are likely to experience distress from pain and other symptoms, and psychosocial concerns. In low-income countries such as Myanmar, Laos, and Cambodia many cancer patients are unable to receive even basic anti-cancer treatment. In these countries, supportive and palliative care is the first choice for economically disadvantaged people (Payne et al., 2012).

Context of health care services and systems

Globally health care systems are often under pressure with competing priorities including; child and maternal health, curative treatment for communicable diseases, or mental health, and often in the context of increasingly constrained financial resources. There are various models of funding for hospices and palliative care such as charitable donations in the United Kingdom, medical insurance reimbursement in the United States (US) government funding such as in

Australia, with many complex mixed models of funding particular aspects of palliative care. This complexity is often a barrier to accessing services, or may mean that Western models are just not transferrable to low- and middle-income countries (Rajagopal and George, 2015). The WHO advocate a Public Health Model based on four components: appropriate national policies, adequate availability of opioids and essential medicines, education of health care workers and the public, and implementation of all levels of palliative care services (Stjernsward et al., 2007). These can be implemented within the context of cultural norms and country-wide resources, with Mongolia providing an example of successful development of hospice facilities and education programmes (The Lien Foundation, 2015).

Palliative care services

Overall there has been a steady growth in the development of palliative care services in most parts of the world (WHO and WPCA 2014; The Lien Foundation, 2015). Access to good quality health services, of which palliative care forms a part, is crucial for the improvement of health outcomes. However, over at least the last decade, it has been increasingly recognized that there are major constraints in health professional workforce capacity. This is partly because of the unbalanced distribution of health professionals between and within countries (Dussault and Franceschini, 2006). In all countries, there are higher proportions of health professionals located in urban and wealthy areas; compounding the disadvantages to poorer and rural populations. For example, while African countries suffer 24 per cent of the global disease burden, they have only 3 per cent of the world's health professional workforce (Collins et al., 2010). In some resource-rich countries, there is inward migration, largely for economic reasons, of physicians who may be trained elsewhere. Likewise, there are similar patterns of migration for nurses and care assistants such as from central and Eastern Europe to Western Europe, or from India and the Philippines to the Middle East. These changes impact upon their families, especially children and older people left behind, and present an enormous obstacle for the delivery of health services in the countries of origin, including building palliative care capacity. In some places volunteers help to fill these gaps as will be illustrated in subsequent chapters.

New opportunities and challenges

This section seeks to identify new opportunities and challenges facing palliative care. It offers insights into what care needs to be provided and potential solutions to the barriers for subsequent developments. We focus specifically on international and national policy initiatives as drivers for change in facilitating the development of palliative care. Nowhere is this more important than in improving access to opioids and essential medicines. However, we continue to see large differences in the availability of pain medications globally, resulting in unnecessary suffering in the final phase of life (Scholten et al., 2014). This links with the need for robust quality indicators to explicitly define measurable items referring to the outcomes, processes, and structure of palliative care. Current quality indicators such as consumption of opioids by cancer patients are inherently flawed by their emphasis merely upon cancer patients and pain relief; while in themselves these are important aspects of palliative care, they fail to encompass psycho-social and spiritual elements of palliative care, and do not address the needs of non-cancer patients for adequate pain relief (Payne et al., 2012). The need to ensure accessible and affordable opioids and essential medicines remains a barrier in many low- and middle-income countries with overly restrictive legislation or clinical protocols (Rajogopal and George, 2015). A recent analysis of legal documents from 11 countries in central and Eastern Europe identified nine categories of potential barriers, ranging from 22 in Cyprus to 128 in Lithuania, to obtaining effective pain control, especially for those with non-cancerous illnesses (Vranken et al., 2014).

Policy developments

One of the most important recent developments to facilitate the widespread adoption of palliative care was the endorsement by the World Health Assembly in May 2014, of a resolution calling for governments to integrate palliative care into national health care systems. Evidence suggests that the development of national policies or strategic plans provides a framework for fostering the growth of services, such as the National Palliative Care Strategy in Australia in 2000 and the End of Life Care Strategy of England and Wales in 2008. In other countries there has been enacted legislation that provides access to palliative care such as home palliative care in Germany (see Chapter 6). One concern has been the focus of strategic plans upon palliative care for people with cancer, when the increasing prevalence of patients with neurodegenerative and chronic conditions means that a wider coverage is warranted. Palliative care clinical tools and pathways need to be developed and rigorously tested to ensure patient and public acceptability and cultural sensitivity to prevent fiascos such as that of the Liverpool Care Pathway (Department of Health, 2013). This was a quality improvement checklist for end-of-life care in hospitals that was withdrawn after a public inquiry identified serious shortcomings in its evidence base and implementation.

A public health approach to palliative care emphasizes the importance of primary care and generalists in up-scaling better symptom management in end-stage conditions. There appears to be an increasing recognition that palliative care should be delivered early in the trajectory and offer opportunities to improve not only physical symptom management but also enhanced communication, psychosocial care, and promote quality of life. An influential study of early integration of palliative care into oncology treatment of patients with lung cancer demonstrated that adding palliative care consultations to standard cancer treatment significantly improved quality of life and increased survival by a few months compared to controls in the United States of America (Temel et al., 2010). A number of initiatives are now being developed to better integrate palliative care into the standard treatment protocols of cancer patients, and to a lesser extent in heart failure, respiratory disease, and other chronic conditions. However, chronic diseases with a more complex or prolonged trajectory at the end of life present more challenges in enabling physicians to identify when to refer to palliative care. There is also a more limited evidence base on the effectiveness of palliative care interventions within these conditions.

Education and training

One of the major challenges threatening the expansion of palliative care is the limitation on workforce capacity. This can be considered in two ways: firstly, in the need to increase the number of health care professionals with sufficient expertise to be regarded as a specialist, and secondly, the need to promote basic understanding of palliative care in all health and social care workers. In many countries, palliative care is not a designated specialist medical discipline, although the numbers of professionals practising in that capacity continue to grow. One of the major challenges for the future is to improve equity of access to good quality care during the final phase of life, however long that may last, not just end-of-life care. It is likely that advances in medicine and health technologies will mean that greater numbers of people will survive for longer with complex health and social care needs. This will mean a different type of workforce is required to provide a basic palliative care approach wherever the patient and family are located, and opportunities for advice, support, and referral to specialist palliative care providers. One option is for specialist palliative care workers to facilitate and coordinate care, rather than provide 'hands-on' care, which means that developing knowledge and skills in consultancy, advocacy, education, and leadership will form essential components alongside excellent knowledge of pain and symptom management, and psychosocial and spiritual support (Payne and Lynch, 2015). In resource-poor countries, it is essential that appropriate, sustainable models are developed, including volunteer workers (Rajogopal and George, 2015).

However, in many countries, undergraduate medical curricula do not include palliative care as a core topic. A recent survey of the 53 countries in the WHO European region indicated that in 14 countries no palliative care was taught, and in only 13 countries was the subject taught in all medical schools (Carrasco et al., 2015). There is, therefore, an urgent need to increase postgraduate training in palliative care and include it in post basic qualifications for those specializing in primary care, oncology, and geriatric medicine. The EAPC have published recommendations on core competences in palliative care for all members of the multidisciplinary team (Gamondi et al., 2013). The provision of similar guidance for volunteers is urgently required.

Implications for volunteering

The chapter ends by providing a short description of a few studies investigating the role of volunteers drawn from the United Kingdom, to illustrate the types of innovative ways that volunteers can be involved in supporting patients and their families as they face advanced disease and the final phase of life.

It is recognized that volunteers make a substantial contribution to the effective delivery of palliative care services. The economic, political, and demographic challenges of the twenty-first century raise many questions about how best to involve volunteers within this specialist setting. Horton Smith (2013) provides evidence that academic interest in studying volunteerism has grown since the 1970s, but specific research into volunteering in palliative care is still patchy and often focuses on the individual traits of volunteers. In addition, the ways in which volunteering is organized across the globe varies considerably, making comparisons and conclusions difficult. However, recent research examples may help to shed some light on the innovative ways in which this invaluable resource can be developed and succoured.

A recent nationwide study in England studied the current picture of volunteer deployment (Burbeck et al., 2014) and then explored in more depth the issues and practices of managing volunteers (Morris et al., 2015). It was noted that volunteer management practice was generally well developed and has become increasingly formalized, with policies and procedures around recruitment, training, support and discipline common. However, specific areas of emotional support and performance management still require development. Moreover, there are dramatic differences in terms of the level and nature of training and support offered to volunteers even in the same roles in different organizations, for example, training varied from only informal and on-the-job to a standardized 24-hour programme for all volunteers. Despite generally robust management practice, the evidence suggests substantial scope for hospices to develop the strategic aspects of their volunteering. Among the potential areas for development were recognizing the role of volunteer management as a profession with a distinctive skill set; expanding the roles of volunteers into direct care and community care whilst recognizing the need for more sophisticated risk management and support mechanisms; increasing the diversity of volunteers; adopting a dual-track approach to developing traditional volunteer roles and embracing newer forms of professionally skilled, output focused roles; facilitating greater co-operation across hospices; and targeting greater community engagement by taking advantage of volunteers' unique position between the hospice setting and the community.

Six local Age UK organizations in England were funded to provide practical and emotional support to older family carers, and to establish the potential role of trained volunteer-delivered interventions in this area (Morbey et al., 2013). An evaluation concluded that it was difficult to recruit volunteers to this rather specialist role, and that they required considerable on-going support to maintain the in-home services. It was recommended that volunteering to support people facing the end of life should be recognized and promoted as a specialist service, whether it is a dedicated service or embedded in a wider organization. End of life volunteering should involve specialist training, contact with peer volunteers working in the same area, and robust mechanisms for supervision and support.

Another study aims to evaluate social action initiatives which use volunteers to deliver befriending services to people anticipated to be in their last year of life. The research used a wait-list randomized controlled trial (WLRCT) and qualitative case study to evaluate 12 hospice and charitable organizations. Patients were randomly allocated to either receive the social action volunteer befriending service straight away or receive the intervention after a four-week wait (wait-list arm). The impact of the intervention on end-of-life experience (quality of life as primary outcome, and loneliness, and social support as secondary outcomes) was measured (Walshe et al., 2016). The trial demonstrated no significant difference in main or secondary outcomes at four weeks. Rate of decrease in quality-of-life scores showed trends in favour of the intervention (Walshe, Dodd et al., 2016).

Conclusions

In this chapter we identified a number of important issues for the provision of specialist volunteer support services for patients and family carers who are nearing the end of life. Well-rehearsed demographic projections indicate burgeoning populations of people needing support and care by volunteers in their homes and communities. There are increasing expectations and demands from the public for improvement to end-of-life care, greater engagement with volunteers is one way to achieve this.

References

Berry, P. and Planalp, S. (2008) Ethical issues for hospice volunteers. *American Journal of Hospice and Palliative Care* **25**(6): 458–62.

Burbeck, R., et al. (2014) Volunteers in specialist palliative care: a survey of adult services in the United Kingdom. *Journal of Palliative Medicine* **17**(5): 568–74.

Carrasco, J.M., et al. (2015) Palliative care medical education in European universities: a descriptive study and numerical scoring system proposal for assessing educational development. *Journal of Pain and Symptom Management* (in press).

Clark, D. (2002) *Cicely Saunders, Founder of the Hospice Movement: Selected Letters 1959–1999.* Oxford: Oxford University Press.

Collins, F.S., Glass, R.I., Whitescarver, J., Wakefield, M., and Goosby, E.P. (2010) Developing health workforce capacity in Africa. *Science* **330**(6009): 1324–5.

Department of Health (2013). *More Care, Less Pathway: A Review of the Liverpool Care Pathway.* London. Available from: https://www.gov.uk/government/uploads/system/uploads/attachment_data/file/212450/Liverpool_Care_Pathway.pdf. Accessed 19 February 2016.

Dussault, G. and Franceschini, M.C. (2006) Not enough there, too many here: understanding geographical imbalances in the distribution of the health workforce. *Human Resources for Health* **4**: 12. doi: 10.1186/1478-4491-4-12.

Field-Richards, S.E. and Arthur, A. (2012) Negotiating the boundary between paid and unpaid hospice workers: a qualitative study of how hospices volunteers understand their work. *American Journal of Hospice and Palliative Medicine.* doi: 10.1177/1049909111435695.

Gamondi, C., Larkin, P., and Payne, S. (2013) Core competencies in palliative care: an EAPC White Paper on palliative care education—Part 1. *European Journal of Palliative Care* **20**(2): 86–91.

Hall, S., Petkova, H., Tsouros, A.D., Costantini, M., and Higginson, I. (2011) *Palliative Care For Older People: Better Practices.* Denmark: World Health Organization.

Horton Smith, D. (2013) Growth of research associations and journals in the emerging discipline of altruistics. *Nonprofit and Voluntary Sector Quarterly* **42**(4): 638–56. doi: 10.1177/0899764013495979.

Humphreys, C. (2001). 'Waiting for the last summons': the establishment of the first hospices in England 1878–1914. *Mortality* **6**: 146–66.

Low J., et al. (2005) A qualitative evaluation of the impact of palliative care day services: the experiences of patients, informal carers, day unit managers and volunteer staff. *Palliative Medicine* **19**(1): 65–70.

McKee, M., Kelley, M.L., and Guirguis-Younger, M. (2007) So no one dies alone: a study of hospice volunteering with rural seniors. *Journal of Palliative Care* **23**(3) 163–72.

Morbey, H., Payne, S., Froggatt, K., Milligan, C., and Turner, M. (2013) *Supporting Older Carers of those Nearing the End of Life: Lancaster University Evaluation of Six Pilot Projects.* Lancaster University, Unpublished report for Age UK.

Morris, S., Wilmot, A., Hill, M., Ockenden, O., and Payne, S. (2013) A narrative literature review of the contribution of volunteers in end-of-life care services. *Palliative Medicine* 27: 428–36.

Morris, S.M., Payne, S., Ockenden, N., and Hill, M. (2015) Hospice volunteers: bridging the gap to the community? *Health and Social Care in the Community*. doi: 10.1111/hsc.12232.

Murtagh, F., Bausewein, C., Verne, J., Groeneveld, E.I., Kaloki, Y., and Higginson, I.J. (2014) How many people need palliative care? A study developing and comparing methods for population-based estimates *Palliative Medicine* 28(1): 49–58.

Payne, S. (2001) The role of volunteers in hospice bereavement support in New Zealand. *Palliative Medicine* 15(2): 107–15.

Payne, S., Chan, N., Davies, A., Poon, E., Connor, S., and Goh, C. (2012) Supportive, palliative, and end-of-life care for patients with cancer in Asia: resource-stratified guidelines from the Asian Oncology Summit 2012. *Lancet Oncology* (13): 492–500.

Payne, S., Leget, C., Peruselli, C., and Radbruch, L. (2012) Quality indicators for palliative care: debates and dilemmas. *Palliative Medicine* 26(5): 679–80.

Payne, S. and Lynch, T. (2015) International progress in creating palliative medicine as a specialized discipline and the development of palliative care. In Cherny, N.I., Fallon, M.T., Kaasa, S., Portenoy, R.K., and Currow, D.C. (eds) *Oxford Textbook of Palliative Care*, 5th edition. Oxford: Oxford University Press, (pp. 3–9).

Radbruch, L., and Payne, S. (2009) White Paper on standards and norms for hospice and palliative care in Europe: part 1. *European Journal of Palliative Care* 16(6): 278–89.

Payne, S. and Radbruch, L. (2010) White Paper on standards and norms for hospice and palliative care in Europe: part 2. *European Journal of Palliative Care* 17(1): 22–33.

Rajogopal, M.R. and George R. (2015) Providing palliative care in economically disadvantaged countries. In Cherny, N.I., Fallon. M.T., Kaasa, S., Portenoy, R.K., and Currow, D.C. (eds) *Oxford Textbook of Palliative Care*, 5th edition. Oxford: Oxford University Press, (pp. 10–18).

Savery, C.A. and Egbert, N. (2010) Hospice volunteer as patient advocate: a trait approach. *Palliative and Supportive Care* 8(2): 159–67. doi: 10.1017/S1478951509990915.

Scholten, W., Payne, S., and Radbruch, L. (2014) Access to opioid medicines in Europe. *Le Courier des addictions* 16(4): 3–4.

Scott, R. (2015). 'We cannot do it without you'- the impact of volunteers in UK hospices. *European Journal of Palliative Care* 22(2): 80–83.

Sepulveda, C., Marlin, A. Yoshida, T., and Ullrich, A. (2002). Palliative care: The World Health Organization's global perspective. *Journal of Pain and Symptom Management* 24(2): 91–6.

Sevigny, A., Dumont, S., Robin Cohen, S., and Frappier A. (2010) Helping them live until they die: volunteer practices in palliative home care. *Nonprofit and Voluntary Sector Quarterly* 39: 734–52. doi: 10.1177/0899764009339074.

Smeding, R. and Mason, S. (2012) OPCARE9 work package 5—the role of volunteers. *European Journal of Palliative Care* 19(3): 124–6.

Stjernsward, J., Foley K., and Ferris F. (2007) The public health strategy for palliative care. *Journal of Pain and Symptom Management* 33(5): 514–20.

Temel, J., et al. (2010) Early palliative care for patients with metastatic non-small-cell lung cancer. *New England Journal of Medicine* **363**: 733–42.

The Lien Foundation (2015) *Quality of Death Index*, 2nd edition. Singapore: The Lien Foundation.

van den Block, L., Albers, G., Pereira, S., Pasman, R., Onwuteaka-Philipsen, B., and Deliens, L. (2015) *Palliative Care for Older People: A Public Health Perspective.* Oxford: Oxford University Press.

Vranken, M., et al. (2014) Legal barriers in accessing opioid medicines: results of the ATOME quick scan of national legislation of Eastern European countries. *Journal of Pain and Symptom Management.* doi: 10.1016/j.jpainsymman.2014.02.013.

Walshe, C., Dodd, S. et al. (2016) How effective are volunteers at supporting people in their last year of life? A pragmatic randomised wait-list trial in palliative care (ELSA). *BMC Medicine* **14**: 203.doi: 10.1186/s12916-016-0746-8.

Walshe, C., et al. (2016) Protocol for the End-of-Life Social Action Study (ELSA): a randomised wait-list controlled trial and embedded qualitative case study evaluation assessing the causal impact of social action befriending services on end of life experience. *BMC Palliative Care* **15**.60. doi:10.1186/s12904-016-0134-3.

Weeks, L.E., et al. (2008) Hospice palliative care volunteers: A Unique Care Link. *Journal of Palliative Care* **24**(2): 85–93.

Woitha, K., et al. (2015) Volunteers in palliative care—a comparison of seven European countries: a descriptive dtudy. *Pain Practice* **15**(6): 572–9.

World Health Organisation and Worldwide Palliative Care Alliance (2014) *Global Atlas of Palliative Care at the End of Life.* New York: WPCA.

Factsheet. World Health Organisation (2016) Available from: www.who.int/mediacentre/factsheet/fs310/en/intex2.html. Accessed 17 February 2016.

Chapter 3

Volunteering in hospice and palliative care in the United Kingdom

Ros Scott

History of hospice and palliative care volunteering in the United Kingdom

Volunteers are an essential part of hospice and palliative care as already highlighted by Payne and Morris in Chapter 2. Radbruch et al. (2010) suggest 'the hospice movement as a civil rights movement, is based on volunteers.' (p. 26). This is certainly true of the United Kingdom (UK) where volunteers are inextricably linked with the history and development of hospice and palliative care. Indeed most voluntary sector hospices were founded by volunteers (Scott, 2015). (Voluntary sector hospices in the UK are those which are largely funded by charitable donations. Different types of hospices and funding are explored more fully later in the chapter). This chapter will explore the UK history and background of volunteering; the scope of involvement; the legislative, regulatory and political influences; approaches to management and training, and how volunteering is changing. The chapter will conclude by exploring the factors that influence the success of volunteering.

Dame Cicely Saunders is recognized as the founder of the modern hospice movement in the UK, and her work has influenced the development of hospice and palliative care services around the world (Clark et al., 2005). Recognizing that her vision for the care of dying people could not be met within the National Health Service (NHS), Dame Cicely set out to establish a different ethos and approach. The culmination of this was the establishment of St Christopher's Hospice in London which opened in 1967. She had experience as a volunteer at St Luke's hospital London (Saunders, 2002). In a letter from Dame Cicely Saunders to Jenny Hunt (Private correspondence, March 2003) she was clear that her intention from the beginning was to ensure that volunteers were integral to the work of hospices to ensure that the hospice 'belonged' to the community. She believed that the way to achieve this was to invite people from the community to share their skills through volunteering in the hospice.

Whilst the word 'hospice' in the UK has become synonymous with hospice buildings, such care is provided in many different settings. In addition to in-patient and day care within the hospice, care is also delivered in the community and in care homes.

Typically the role and influence of volunteers in voluntary sector hospice and palliative care services changes depending on the stage of development of the organization (Scott, 2013). In the founding stages of the organization, it is volunteers within the local community who drive the idea forward often taking it from a concept to reality, through lobbying for the provision of services, fundraising, and even commissioning the hospice building. Once paid staff are employed, the position and influence of volunteers changes from leadership to a supporting role. The exception to this is the hospice board comprised entirely of volunteers in their role as trustees. The board has a collective responsibility for the strategic direction of their organization, ensuring that all legal obligations and regulatory requirements are met, and that resources are used effectively. The board also provides line management to the chief executive, who has delegated responsibility for the effective management of the hospice. As trustees, there-fore, volunteers play an important role and carry significant legal obligations. Often not recognized as volunteers, Turner and Payne (2008) suggest that there is a need for a better understanding of these 'hidden' volunteers.

The children's hospice movement emerged much later with the opening of the first UK children's hospice, Helen House in Oxford, in 1982. Children's hospices were founded in the main by religious organizations or by families of a child with a life-threatening/life-limiting condition who identified a gap in provision of much-needed care and support. Children's hospices, however, took longer than their adult counterparts to embrace the concept of volunteering (Scott, 2009). The reasons given for this included the complexity of the children's conditions, the large number of professionals already involved in the lives of these families, and concerns about safeguarding. However, as the benefits of volunteering were recognized following the experiences of a few pioneering services, this has steadily grown. Almost every voluntary sector children's hos-pice now involves volunteers in some capacity, (Carling and Howlett, 2013) and volunteers are also involved within a number of voluntary sector and NHS paediatric palliative care teams.

Scope of volunteer involvement

Hospices rely on volunteering to enable them to deliver the range and quality of services on which those they care for depend (Davis Smith, 2004; Sallnow, 2010; Radbruch et al., 2010). Research suggests that there is a strong link be-tween volunteers and the sustainability of voluntary sector hospices, and that some would undoubtedly have to close without the involvement of volunteers (Scott, 2015).

It is estimated that there are approximately 160,000 volunteers in the UK giving around 23 million hours of time every year, in both adult and children's hospices (Scott, 2015). Whilst the difference volunteers make to organizations is significant in terms of the time and skills that they bring, their impact on patients and families and their influence in helping organizations to achieve their goals, their value in financial terms may also be calculated. Based on these figures, it is estimated that this represents an economic value of approximately £150 m (Scott, 2015).

We have already seen that volunteers play a key role in the governance of voluntary sector hospice and palliative care services, however, these trustee roles would not be found within equivalent NHS services. Typically within voluntary sector hospices, volunteers are involved in inpatient units, day care, and home care. Volunteers are also involved in NHS hospices, some NHS palliative care wards, and community teams, and can now also to be found in some care homes for older people.

Within these different settings volunteers undertake a diverse range of roles. (Scott, 2015; Burbeck et al., 2014). For the purposes of this chapter these have been grouped and summarized under three main categories: 1) direct support (practical, social, and emotional) to patients and their families, 2) organizational support, and 3) income generation and community awareness raising.

Direct support

Direct support for patients and families includes practical, social, and emotional support. Examples of practical support include: shopping, gardening, housework, caring for pets, providing transport for patients and families, taking patients out, and helping patients to engage with hobbies and activities.

Social and emotional support encompasses a range of volunteer roles. These might include spending time with patients and their carers, talking/listening to their anxieties and concerns, and sitting with patients at end of life, creative activities and therapies, complementary therapies, beauty therapy and hairdressing, counselling, pastoral and spiritual care, bereavement support, information giving, gathering patient feedback, and support with physiotherapy and occupational therapy (Burbeck et al., 2014).

In children's hospices direct support might additionally include: art and music activities, befriending for parents and carers, befriending for young people, play activities with affected children and their siblings, and providing bereavement support to families (Burbeck et al., 2013).

Organizational support

Organizational support describes the help given by volunteers within hospice buildings and grounds. Within adult and children's services this typically includes: reception duties, administrative support, helping with housekeeping, helping in the kitchen, serving meals and refreshments, providing home baking, gardening, help with odd jobs, and maintenance.

Income generation and awareness raising

Local voluntary sector hospices not only provide the majority of hospice care throughout the UK, but also contribute significant levels of funding (Hospice UK and Together for Short Lives, 2015). Adult hospices receive less than 33 per cent of funding from government sources, and for children's hospices this figure is even lower, at around 17 per cent (Hospice UK, 2016). A recent survey of adult and children's hospices suggested that such funding was at best static, and at worst falling (Hospice UK and Together for Short Lives, 2015). This means that voluntary sector hospices must raise in excess of two thirds of the funds required to run their services by fundraising. It is estimated that collectively such hospices in the UK have to raise around £2.7 million every day from their local communities. This is what sets the UK aside from a number of other countries (Ellershaw, 2015) and explains why there are so many more volunteers involved in fundraising activities than in supporting patients and families. Volunteers are involved in a wide range of income generation activities to support the fundraising staff. This includes running local fundraising groups, giving talks to different community organizations about the work of the hospice, organizing or working at events or undertaking collections, helping with fundraising administration, and writing thank you letters to donors. For many hospice and palliative care organizations in the UK, charity shops are an important source of income. These depend heavily on volunteer support to enable them to function, with some relying solely on volunteers to manage and run shops.

Another important aspect of the role of volunteers in both voluntary and statutory hospice and palliative care services is the strong link that they bring to the local community. Morris et al. (2015) suggest that hospices are sometimes seen as inward-looking organizations, connecting mainly with others in the hospice and palliative care field. Volunteers, as members of the local community, offer a channel of communication both bringing community views into the organization and helping to inform the community about the work of the hospice (Morris et al., 2015). This awareness raising contributes significantly to educating the public in palliative and end of life care and breaking down taboos, which helps to make hospices more accessible (Scott, 2015). However, hospices could do so much more to purposefully improve the diversity of their volunteers, and develop their educational role (Morris et al., 2015).

The legislative and political influences

The effects of legislation, regulation, and policy can have a significant effect on volunteering, either directly or indirectly. Volunteers and volunteering are not defined in law within the UK. Anecdotal evidence suggests that views are divided about whether this is a positive situation allowing volunteering to flourish without interference, or whether this denies volunteer rights and fair treatment. Despite this lack of specific legislation, laws introduced for other purposes have consequences for hospice and palliative care volunteering. Examples of this include Health and Safety and employment legislation, and the requirement for criminal record checking for all people who wish to be employed, or volunteer in certain roles with children or vulnerable adults. This can make it challenging for organizations and volunteer managers, who have to ensure that volunteering works within the framework of certain laws, without contravening others. For example, organizations have to ensure that their approach to and documentation on volunteering does not constitute a contract of employment in law. If this were to be the case, volunteers would be entitled to all the rights of an employee, including being paid the minimum wage.

Hospice and palliative care services also exist within a regulated framework with which volunteering must comply. The standards against which hospice and palliative care services are inspected often do not specifically refer to volunteering, however, there tends to be an implicit expectation that, where standards relate to staff, that these also apply to volunteers (Scott, 2014).

From a political perspective, and as already discussed in more detail in Chapter 1, successive UK governments have sought to promote volunteering. One key example is the 'Big Society' (Cabinet Office, 2010) initiative, intended to increase the levels of volunteering within the UK (discussed in more detail by Howlett in Chapter 1). This brought a drive towards voluntary organizations undertaking work, previously delivered by statutory organizations, and the move to more formalized volunteering. One consequence of this policy is an increased demand for volunteering, at a time when individuals have many competing demands on their time (Guild et al., 2014). There is no doubt that the political environment in the UK is one that is keen to promote the development of volunteering. However, within a climate of economic austerity in recent years, this is not matched by the necessary funding to facilitate such development (Guild et al., 2014).

Alongside this there has also been an almost unprecedented focus on palliative care in recent years, during which time, a number of significant policies have been developed in the four countries of the UK, Scotland, England, Wales, and Northern Ireland. The intent of these policies is to ensure that all those with palliative care needs receive appropriate care, regardless of diagnosis. Volunteering is largely overlooked by many of these policies, which is of concern given the level of dependence on volunteering for the delivery of services.

Approaches to management

Hospice and palliative care organizations are typically supported by many hundreds of volunteers, each with a specific role. Generally, there is a clear structure with overall management of the voluntary service from a volunteer manager, with local line management by paid staff in the relevant area of work. Hospice volunteering models in this country would generally be considered as 'formal' volunteering, as described by Rochester et al. (2010). Describing this as the dominant paradigm, it is typified by organizations involving volunteers for the purpose of delivering a service to others. Volunteers usually work within a hierarchical structure, with clearly designated boundaried roles, and are managed by paid staff. Critics of this model suggest that it is not sustainable, appropriate for, or compatible with today's volunteers. Indeed it is suggested that while the journey towards the professionalization of volunteering may benefit hospices in terms of clarity of boundaries and management, but that this has a disadvantageous effect on the experience of volunteers and their subsequent relationship with patients (Guirguis-Younger et al., 2005). This presents volunteer managers with the challenge of maximizing the role of and ethos of volunteering, diversifying volunteer teams in line with local needs, and meeting formal regulatory requirements (Morris et al., 2013).

Standards and training

Quality and safety are important components of volunteering. Within the UK there are no specific palliative care volunteering standards, however, many organizations have successfully achieved the national quality standard Investing in Volunteers (IiV, n.d.). This is a generic, national quality standard for volunteering and there are a number of other such standards available to organizations. General standards for volunteer management in the UK (Skills-Third Sector, 2010) provide a framework for management competencies. Some hospices refer to these when developing or reviewing volunteer manager job descriptions.

Whilst there are many general training courses available for volunteer managers, including an undergraduate degree course, there is no specialised, accredited training for volunteer managers in palliative care. However, there is a national professional association, the Association of Voluntary Service Managers (AVSM, n.d.) which promotes best practice and the sharing of knowledge and experience within the field.

All hospice and palliative care volunteers in the UK undertake training. However as Payne and Morris suggest in Chapter 2, the content and structure of this training depends on the local service, and on the role undertaken by the volunteer. Whilst training programmes may differ from organization to organization, they many commonly include topics such as: an introduction to the organization; the principles of palliative care, the needs of patients and families; understanding death, dying and bereavement, the role of the volunteer, responsibilities and boundaries, and self-care. In addition volunteers must undertake statutory mandatory training such as health and safety, moving and handling, infection control, and more specific training relating to the role. However, it must be noted that little research evidence exists to underpin the content of programmes or to evaluate their efficacy.

A national training framework and competencies are currently being piloted for children's palliative care volunteers in the community.

Why and how volunteering in this field is changing

We have seen in Chapter 2 how hospice and palliative care is changing from an international perspective. In common with many countries, the UK has an aging population. This is expected to cause a significant increase in the demand for hospice and palliative care services in the future as people live longer with increasingly complex long-term conditions (Calanzani et al., 2013). Inevitably this will have considerable implications for volunteering as hospices respond to the changing needs and demands of patients and their families. Naylor et al. (2013) suggest that within the current health and social care context that 'it is more important than ever to think strategically about the role of volunteering. The health and social care system will find it increasingly difficult to meet its objectives without doing so' (p. viii).

As discussed in more detail in Chapter 1, volunteering is also changing. With societal changes, more women are now working, there is an increase in single parent families and single people households, grandparents are now frequently the main source of child care for working parents, young people at college and university must work to support themselves through their studies and many face a future with student debt. Added to the many choices that people have for spending their leisure time, this means that people have less time available to volunteer. A growing older population could present many opportunities for volunteering, at the same time as improving the health and wellbeing of volunteers. However, changes to pensions in the UK mean that many people are now working longer, with some struggling to afford to retire. Volunteers in the future may not be able to make such regular or long-term commitments as in the past, and they rightly have high expectations of how their time and skill are used (Guild et al., 2014).

With the rise of a new generation of volunteers with greater demands on their time and higher expectations of volunteering, it is likely that the era of the volunteer committed to giving time every week indefinitely, is coming to an end. This, therefore, poses challenges for the sector where volunteers are involved in supporting patients and families and for whom ongoing relationships and continuity is important. In recent years, however, there has been much discussion about the advantages and disadvantages of the traditional 'lifetime volunteer'. It has been suggested that there may be benefits of a time-limited approach to recruitment, both to the organization and the volunteer. This approach may make volunteering more accessible to and compatible with the expectations of the 'new volunteer'. It may also prevent the 'institutionalization' of volunteers, who over time may become resistant to change (as discussed more fully by Hartley in Chapter 13). However, this would not preclude longer-term volunteering where, following regular review, commitment may be renewed as long as the relationship remains mutually beneficial.

Despite changes in volunteering, hospice and palliative care services, in the main, still seem to attract and retain volunteers without too much difficulty. This is likely to be a reflection of their strong relationships with their local communities. Many hospice volunteers have been touched by the service and are keen to give something back. Anecdotal evidence suggests, however, that increasing numbers of volunteers are required to maintain the same level of services as in previous years as people offer less-regular commitment. Services, therefore, must be alert to the fluctuations in volunteering and plan for volunteering as part of their strategy.

A changing approach to the management of volunteering in hospice and palliative care services in the UK has emerged in recent years. Increasingly, old models of volunteer management, where the volunteer manager was responsible for all volunteers ('my volunteers') has given way to the recognition that not only was this unsustainable, but that for volunteering to be successful, it needed to become everybody's business (Scott, 2014). What has emerged is a model where volunteers are more integrated and paid staff are responsible for the volunteers with whom they work. The volunteer manager, as the professional expert in volunteering, provides support and guidance to the organization at all levels, and to staff and volunteers (Scott, 2014).

Recommendations resulting from the Commission into the Future of Hospice Care (Help the Hospices, 2012) suggested that volunteers are vital to the future of hospice services, and that their contributions could be further extended. The report calls for volunteers to become fully integrated into clinical teams to provide more direct support to patients and families, not only in hospice services, but also in the community.

Anecdotal evidence suggests that volunteers in recent years have become increasingly involved in the direct support of patients and their families. Whilst volunteers have historically been involved in in-patient wards and day-care settings, the greatest change has been volunteers providing support to patients and families in the community in both the adult and children's palliative care sectors.

The Marie Curie Helper Service is one example of this. Marie Curie volunteers known as 'Helpers' provide practical, social, and emotional support to terminally ill patients and their carers by visiting them in their homes on a weekly basis (Marie Curie Helper, 2011). Apart from providing companionship to patients, Helpers undertake every-day practical household tasks; help patients and families to find advice and also escort patients on outings or to social events. They also provide respite to carers enabling them to have time to do what is important to them (for example being able to attend appointments or visit the hairdresser). An evaluation of the service undertaken in 2011 found that the support offered by the Helpers made a significant difference to terminally ill people and their families. Patients and carers reported a positive impact on their emotional health and wellbeing (Prentice et al., 2013).

The increasing development of volunteering in the community has given volunteers more autonomy in how they work (even in the more formal context), enabling them to respond to the individual needs of patients and families as they arise, within the agreed boundaries of their role. Although in many cases volunteers still report to paid staff, there are a growing number of examples of volunteer-led projects. This is a significant move away from the restrictive, strictly defined roles of the past. This appears to have been influenced by the growing recognition of the importance of community engagement and of public health approaches to palliative and end of life care as discussed by Sallnow and Richardson in Chapter 14.

One example of a volunteer-led service includes the Hospice Neighbours service at St Nicholas Hospice Care in Suffolk, England. This aims to build community capacity at end of life and is based on health promotion principles. People in the last phase of their lives and their families are matched with volunteers living in the same community, known as 'hospice neighbours'. Over 150 volunteers provide companionship to help to reduce isolation and practical support such as gardening, taking people out, and helping with pets. Local volunteers act as coordinators of the service managing small groups of volunteers, matching volunteers with patients and families and providing volunteers with support. Overall management is provided by a Hospice Neighbours Manager, Coordinator and Administrator. The organization has offered resources and support to other hospice and palliative care services wishing to set up similar services (Barry and Patel, 2013).

Children's hospice and palliative care

This change is also mirrored in the children's palliative care sector, where volunteers increasingly provide practical and emotional support to families who have a child with a life-threatening/life-limiting condition. This shift in volunteering in children's palliative care may be in response to the growing recognition of the needs of families for additional support at home.

In addition to established volunteering within children's hospice and palliative care services, two pilot projects have been conducted in the UK to assess the value of volunteers providing support to families in the community. Evaluation of the first pilot with two children's hospices found that families reported the support from volunteers as invaluable and their sense of wellbeing had improved. A subsequent second pilot in 2016/2017 extended the work beyond hospice services to include voluntary sector and NHS community paediatric palliative care services. The second pilot also aimed to review and test a package of resource materials, including a competency framework and training programme, Entitled "Together We Can", these are now widely available (Together for Short Lives). This will hopefully encourage and enable more services throughout the UK to offer volunteer support to families with a child with a life-threatening/life-limiting condition. Early learning emerging from the second pilot, suggests that the project was beneficial in providing valuable additional support to families, helping to reduce isolation and stress. Volunteers report finding the role both rewarding and challenging, enabling them to develop confidence and skills.

Factors that contribute to success

There are many factors that contribute to the success of volunteering and these can be considered from both organizational and volunteer perspectives.

Participants in a survey of hospice and palliative care services (Scott, 2014) identified a range of factors contributing to the success of volunteering in care. It was recognized that a commitment to the involvement of volunteers, at a strategic level from the board and senior management team, were essential from an organizational perspective. Also highlighted was the importance of training staff in working effectively with volunteers. Other success factors included:

- Good training, including effective induction
- Staff acceptance and understanding of volunteering and effective engagement with volunteers
- Roles, boundaries, and expectations about which everyone is clear
- Effective support and supervision from staff and also from experienced volunteers
- Effective recruitment, selection, and matching to make sure that the right volunteers with the right skills were in the right roles
- The commitment and personality of the volunteer
- Effective supervision from staff
- Effective integration with the professional team
- Clear structures and policies
- Effective management
- Valuing and empowering volunteers to use their skills' (p. 16)

Additional factors identified by a number of different projects outwith this survey included:

- Ensuring that volunteer roles are meeting a clearly identified need
- Involving families, staff, and volunteers in the development of roles
- Shared leadership of volunteering
- Understanding and valuing volunteers' strengths and needs
- Experienced volunteers to mentor others
- Effective governance

Community projects identified key success factors as:

- Flexibility in responding to local and individual need
- Local coordination and strong partnership links
- Local/community responsibility for management of volunteers

Volunteering can only be successful if volunteers remain fulfilled by their volunteering experience and are fully engaged with the service. Anecdotal evidence suggests that factors that contribute to success from a volunteer perspective include:

- Skills are used effectively in meaningful roles, not squandering their time and talents
- Knowing that they make a difference

- Effective communication, training and ongoing support
- A belief in the work of the organization
- Feeling valued as individuals and respected for their skills
- Feeling part of something—a sense of belonging
- Having responsibility and the ability to use their judgement
- Having opportunities for personal and professional development
- Engagement with patients and families in identifying new ways for volunteers to support them

Conclusion

This chapter has explored the history, development, and changing face of volunteering in hospice and palliative care in the UK. It is clear that volunteers have played a significant role in the history and development of hospice and palliative care. As both hospice and palliative care and volunteering continue to change and develop, so too the role of volunteers evolves. Today, volunteers are becoming more involved in supporting patients and families in the community, are more empowered, and the emergence of volunteer-led services is growing. Volunteering is seen as a key resource in enabling hospices to meet the increasing demand for services, both now and in the future. With the rise of a new generation of volunteers, hospice and palliative care services must consider the aspirations of prospective volunteers in tandem with the needs of the organization. It is no longer enough to assume that volunteers of the future will automatically wish to work in the ways of volunteers of the past.

References

AVSM. Available from: http://www.avsm.co.uk

Barry, V., and Patel, M., (2013) *An Overview Of Compassionate Communities In England.* Tipton: Murray Hall Community Trust and London: National Council for Dying Matters.

Burbeck, R., et al. (2014) Volunteers in specialist palliative care: A survey of adult services in the United Kingdom. *Journal of Palliative Medicine.* **17**(5): 568–74. doi: 10.1089/jpm.2013.0157.

Burbeck, R., et al. (2013) Volunteer activity in specialist paediatric palliative care: a national survey. *BMJ Supportive & Palliative Care* 0: 1–7. doi: 10.1136/bmjspcare-2012- 000355.

Cabinet Office, (2010) *Building The Big Society.* Available from:http://www.cabinetoffice.gov.uk

Calanzani, N., Higginson, I.J., Gomes, B. (2013) *Current And Future Needs For Hospice Care: An Evidence-Based Report.* London: Help the Hospices.

Carling, R., and Howlett, S. (2013) Shining a Spotlight on Children's Hospice Volunteers: Report of a Survey Conducted for Together for Short Lives. Bristol: Together for Short Lives.

Clark, D. et al. (2005) *A Bit Of Heaven For The Few? An Oral History Of The Modern Hospice Movement In The United Kindgom.* Lancaster: Observatory Publications.

Davis-Smith, J. (2004) *Volunteering In UK Hospices: Looking To The Future.* London: Help the Hospices.

Ellershaw, J., (2015) Some Context Around Palliative Care In UK, And Aspects Of Volunteering Linked With That. In: **L. Radbruch**, M. Hesse, L. Pelttari, and R. Scott (eds), *The full range of volunteering. Views on palliative care volunteering from seven countries as gathered in March 2014 in Bonn, Germany.* 31 March–4 April 2014, pp. 27–37.

Guirguis-Younger, M., Kelley, M., and McKee, M. (2005). Professionalization of hospice volunteer practices: what are the implications? *Palliative and Supportive Care* 3(2), 143–4.

Guild, M., Harrison, T., and Saxton., J. (2014) *The new alchemy. How volunteering turns donations of time and talent into human gold. Part 1, nfp Synergy.* Available from: http://nfpsynergy.net

Help the Hospices, (2012) *Volunteers: vital to the future of hospice care. A working paper of the commission into the future of hospice care.* London: Help the Hospices.

Hospice UK (2016) *Hospice Care in the UK 2016: Scope scale and opportunities.* London: Hospice UK.

Hospice UK and Together for Short Lives (2015) *Commissioning and statutory funding arrangements for hospices in England; Survey results.* London: Hospice UK and Bristol: Together for Short Lives.

Investing in Volunteers Standard. Available from: http://IiV.investinginvolunteers.org.uk/

Marie Curie Helper. (2011) Available from: https://www.mariecurie.org.uk/globalassets/media/documents/how-to-refer-patients/marie-curie-helper-overview.pdf

Morris, S. et al. (2013) A narrative literature review of the contribution of volunteers in end of life care services. *Palliative Medicine.* **27**(5): 428–36. doi: 10.1177/0269216312453608.

Morris, S., Payne, S., Ockenden, N., and Hill, M. (2015) Hospice Volunteers: Bridging the gap to the community? *Health and Social Care in the Community.* doi: 10.1111/hsc.12232.

Naylor, C., Mundle, C., Weaks, L., and Buck, D. (2013) *Volunteering In Health And Care: Securing A Sustainable Future.* London: The Kings Fund.

Prentice, T., et al. (2013) An evaluation of the Marie Curie Helper Service. *BMJ Supportive and Palliative Care* 3(1): 133. doi: 10.1136/bmjspcare-2013-000453b.24.

Private Correspondence between Dame Cicely Saunders and Jenny Hunt. March 2003.

Radbruch, L., and Payne, S. (2010) White Paper On Standards And Norms For Hospice And Palliative Care In Europe Part 2: Recommendations From The European Association For Palliative Care. *European Journal of Palliative Care.* **17**(1): 22–33.

Saunders, C., (2002) in D., Doyle, (ed.) *Volunteers In Hospice And Palliative Care: A Handbook For Volunteer Service Managers.* Oxford: Oxford University Press.

Sallnow, L., (2010) *Conceptualisation of Volunteering in Palliative Care.* MSc Dissertation, Kings College London.

Scott, R., (2009) Volunteers In A Children's Hospice. In: **R. Scott**, S. Howlett, and D. Doyle (eds), *Volunteers In Hospice And Palliative Care: A Resource For Voluntary Services Managers,* 2nd edn. Oxford: Oxford University Press, (pp. 145–59).

Scott, R., (2013) *Strategic Asset Or Optional Extra? The Impact Of Volunteers On Hospice Sustainability.* Doctoral Thesis, University of Dundee.

Scott, R., (2014) *Volunteering: Vital To Our Future How To Make The Most Of Volunteering In Palliative Care.* London: Together for Short Lives: Bristol and Help the Hospices. Available from: www.togetherforshortlives.org.uk or www.hospiceuk.org

Scott R, (2015) We cannot do it without you—the impact of volunteers in UK hospices. *European Journal of Palliative Care* **22**(2): 80–3.

Skills—Third Sector (2010) *Volunteer Managers National Occupational Standards: Pocket-sized edition.* Skills—Third Sector: Sheffield. Available from: http://www. skillsothirdsector.org.uk/documents/NOS_Volunteer_Managers_Pocket_Booklet_ AW3.pdf. Together We Can. Available from http://www.togetherforshortlives.org.uk /news/11952_together_we_can

Turner, M., and **Payne, S.** (2008). Uncovering the hidden volunteers in palliative care: a survey of hospice trustees in the United Kingdom. *Palliative Medicine* **22**(8): 973–4.

Chapter 4

Volunteering in hospice and palliative care in Austria

Leena Pelttari and Anna H. Pissarek

Brief history of palliative care volunteering in Austria

Pioneers in Austria started the first initiatives to improve end of life care in the late 1970s. They were inspired by the work of Dame Cicely Saunders, developments in other European countries, and the significant need for adequate support and care for seriously ill and dying patients in Austria. Among these pioneers was Hildegard Teuschl CS of the congregation of Caritas Socialis Sisters (CS). Her initial approach to hospice work was to start with adequate training and so the first course for volunteers was organized 1979 in Vienna. In other parts of Austria similar courses with the same curriculum were organized by other pioneers. Many participants went back to their federal state or profession and started the first hospice activities. This was the beginning of the development of the Austrian Hospice movement, which began as a voluntary-based movement in all nine federal states.

Realizing that the resources available would not be enough for an inpatient hospice, Caritas, the nonprofit charity organization of the Catholic Church of Austria, founded a mobile team to support seriously ill and dying people at home as the first hospice service in 1989 located in Vienna. Doctors and nurses were all working on a voluntary basis. The team started to grow and today is one of the largest home palliative care support teams in Austria. With a paid multi-professional staff it works in close cooperation with a team of hospice and palliative care volunteers. In 1992 the first Austrian palliative care unit was established, also in Vienna, which was actually an inpatient hospice at that time and was later turned into a palliative care unit for financial reasons.

Hospice Austria, the national independent umbrella organization for hospice and palliative care institutions, was founded in 1993 by Hildegard Teuschl and a group of supporters. As the first president of Hospice Austria and the founder of Master of Palliative Care (MSc) Program she was the most important pioneer of the hospice movement in Austria.

During the last 20 years many teams and structures have been built in different parts of the country. Hospice Austria has developed Austrian standards for volunteers and volunteer managers, curricula for their training and has influenced the development to the stage it has achieved today. The nationwide data survey—conducted annually since 2005—provides an excellent insight into hospice and palliative care in Austria, including volunteering.

In 2015 Austria had 3,630 Hospice and Palliative Care volunteers, people with different backgrounds, different motivations, different life experiences, different ages, and most of them (87 per cent) were female. All volunteers in Austria have to qualify for the challenges that they face in hospice work. Of the total number of volunteers 3,462 belonged to one of the 160 hospice teams and 168 volunteers were working within coordinating organizations (for example, board members and fundraising).

The volunteers contributed in total 405,088 hours (see Figure 4.1). 257,510 (64 per cent) of these were spent in direct patient care, by being with the patient and his/her family, sitting at the bedside, talking or reading to him/her, and doing little errands. The great majority of the volunteers work in cooperation with the other specialized hospice and palliative care services, but they have also started to work in primary care organizations like nursing homes. It will still take some time before hospice and palliative care volunteers are broadly working in general hospitals apart from palliative care units.

Time spent by hospice volunteers in 2015

(Austria overall: 405.088 hours)

CR: 93%

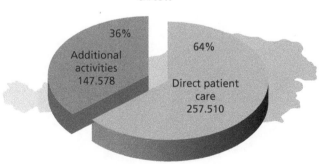

"additional activities" refers to volunteers' supervision and training, volunteers' activities in fundraising, counseling, administrative tasks... as well as the 31.185 hours spent at the regional hospice and palliative care organizations in the 9 federal states of Austria.

Figure 4.1 Hours spent by hospice volunteers in 2015

The number of patients who have been cared for by the voluntary hospice teams has grown significantly during the last 20 years. In 2015 hospice volunteers took care of 12,832 patients. Volunteers also care for the patients' families and those close to them, however, these are excluded from this number. Figure 4.2 shows the places where volunteers offer their care: 26 per cent were at the patients' homes, 13 per cent in general hospital wards, 22 per cent in nursing homes, 31 per cent in specialized palliative care units, so volunteers are working in all palliative care settings. The low number within inpatient hospices—only 4 per cent—is because Austria has only nine inpatient hospices in three out of nine federal states (see Figure 4.2). The reason for this is lack of funding. Palliative care units, on the other hand, are specialized hospital wards that are part of the Austrian health care system with clear public funding. Quite a few of these palliative care units, especially in Vienna, have their 'own' hospice team which accounts for the high percentage of palliative care units as places of care.

In 2009 Hospice Austria organized the first Symposium for Volunteering at the European Association for Palliative Care (EAPC) World Congress in Vienna. This was the beginning of the Austrian involvement in volunteering at a European level. Since then, European symposia have been organized at the EAPC Congresses in Lisbon 2011 and in Prague 2013. The Prague Symposium 'Colourful Life of Hospice Volunteers' was also the starting point for the EAPC

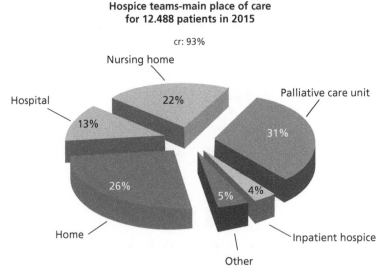

**Hospice teams-main place of care
for 12.488 patients in 2015**

cr: 93%

Nursing home

Hospital

Palliative care unit

22%

13%

31%

26%

5% 4%

Home

Inpatient hospice

Other

Figure 4.2 Hospice teams, main place of care 2015
Copyright © Hospice Austria 2015

Task Force on Hospice and Palliative Care Volunteering in Europe. In 2015 Leena Pelttari (Austria) and Ros Scott (UK), as co-chairs of the EAPC Task Force, organized the 2nd Symposium 'Colourful Life of Hospice Volunteers in Europe', with 160 multi-professional participants from 12 European countries, in Vienna. These symposia have also had a very positive influence on Austrian hospice and palliative care volunteer work. It is very important to learn from experiences in other countries and to get new ideas. The symposia have also been a great motivation for further developments of volunteering in Austria.

Legislative and political influences

There is no specific law for hospice and palliative care volunteering in Austria, but there are some recommendations made by the Ministry of Health and Hospice Austria, as the independent national umbrella organization.

The most important recommendation is the 'Graded Hospice and Palliative Care System' (see Table 4.1). This three-level system was commissioned by the Ministry of Health and developed by Österreichisches Bundesinstitut für Gesundheitswesen (GÖG/ÖBIG), a national research and planning institute for health care in joint cooperation with Hospice Austria in 2004 (Gesundheit Österreich, 2014).

The first level is the primary health care setting with hospitals, nursing homes, and home care. The second level is support care provided by specialists and involves hospital palliative care support teams and home palliative care

Table 4.1 Graded hospice and palliative care system

Hospice and Palliative Care services in Austria				
Primary Care		**Specialised Hospice and Palliative Care**		
	Providers of General Care	**Counseling and support**		**Care**
Acute inpatient care	hospitals	Volunteer Hospice teams	Hospital Palliative Care Support Teams	Palliative Care Units
Long term care	Nursing Homes		Home Palliative Care Support Teams	Inpatient Hospices
Outpatient Care	GP, Therapists, Home Care Services ...			Day Hospices
	Routine Situations 80–90% cases of death	Complex situations, difficult decision making 10–20% cases of death		

Copyright © Hospice Austria and GÖG/ÖBIG 2004

support teams. At the third level, specialized hospice and palliative care is provided in palliative care units, inpatient hospices, and day hospices. Hospice volunteers work as teams in all these contexts. Although the graded system has been integrated into the Austrian Health Care Structure Plan as a recommendation, only the standards for palliative care units are compulsory. However, these standards cover the range of professions, the number and qualifications of staff, and the range and quality of services and infrastructure for all specialized hospice and palliative care organizations. Volunteer Hospice Teams are a very important part of this system as they also cooperate with other services. This system has also become an EAPC recommendation (Radbruch et al., 2009). There is also a separate graded system for children and young adults (Nemeth and Pochobradsky, 2013).

Figure 4.3 shows the development of hospice and palliative care institutions in Austria over the last 20 years. The biggest growth is in volunteer hospice teams. One of the most important reasons for this growth is the cost-effectiveness of hospice volunteer teams compared to other specialized hospice and palliative care institutions. The other reason for the growth is the significant support from Savings Bank Group and Erste Foundation to voluntary hospice teams throughout Austria for almost the last ten years.

In 2014 a Parliamentary Commission of Enquiry for 'Dignity at the end of life' was set up in the Austrian Parliament (Parliamentary Commission for

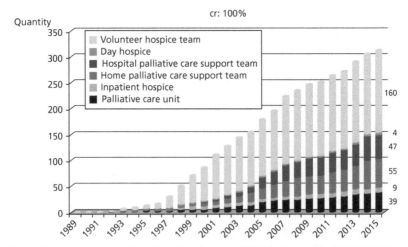

Figure 4.3 Development of Austrian hospice and palliative care services 1989–2015
Copyright © Hospice Austria 2015

Enquiry, 2014). Four days of the Commission's enquiry were discussions open to the public. The concluding report with its 51 recommendations was accepted by all political parties unanimously. Many of these recommendations recognize and include hospice and palliative care volunteers as an integral part of hospice and palliative care.

Following one of the recommendations the Austrian government established a Hospice and Palliative Care Forum in May 2016 in order to promote the development of hospice and palliative care in Austria. The forum consists of all major national institutions involved in organizing and financing hospice and palliative care including the Ministry of Health, Ministry of Social Affairs, Ministry of Finances, representation from the Federal States, Social insurance, and Hospice Austria. Four major task areas have been defined with one of them being the support of hospice and palliative volunteering which is a welcome development.

As previously mentioned, Hospice Austria and the EAPC Task Force on Volunteering in Hospice and Palliative Care in Europe organized the 2nd European volunteering Symposium in Vienna. As this Symposium was partially financed by the Ministry of Social Affairs, and with the Minister himself stating in his opening speech the importance of voluntary hospice and palliative care work for the whole society as a sign of humanity and solidarity, it is a further indication of volunteering in palliative care being recognized. For many volunteers this was an important sign of public appreciation of their work.

Approaches to management and training

In the very beginning volunteers were mostly working on their own in inpatient hospices and home palliative care support teams. However, they are now organized in Hospice Teams. With the introduction of the graded hospice and palliative care system in 2004 a Hospice Team was defined as a group of 10–20 volunteers qualified according to the curriculum of Hospice Austria with a (paid) coordinator (0.5 full-time equivalent) (Gesundheit Österreich, 2014). Coordinators must have a professional qualification such as nursing or social work in addition to a further multi-professional palliative care course (160 hours with 40 hours practice). Additional requirements of the Hospice Austria nationwide standards require volunteers to participate in team meetings, receive supervision, and undertake ongoing training (at least eight hours per year) (Hospiz Österreich 2008). Volunteers are also required to keep good basic records of their work as Hospice Teams also contribute to the annual data survey by Hospice Austria. Data collected includes the hours volunteers spend in direct patient care and those spent in other activities, how many patients they cared for, where care was given, the age and sex of the patients, and how many people received bereavement support.

Every hospice team is a part of an organization (e.g. Caritas, Red Cross, local Hospice Association, Diakonie, inpatient hospice) which provides accident insurance, reimbursement of travelling and telephone costs, or other expenses that volunteers incur. The organization also provides opportunities for training and further education. The concept of the graded hospice and palliative care system suggests at least one team per 40,000 inhabitants in Austria. These numbers have been updated in 2014 to one team for 30,000—40,000 inhabitants. According to this revised plan Austria would need around 210 hospice teams. In 2015 there were 160 teams equaling coverage of about 76 per cent. In reality, the size of the teams varies considerably, between five and 80 volunteers can make up one team.

In addition to the Hospice Austria Standards for volunteers and volunteer managers there is a manual describing processes for volunteer hospice teams in the graded hospice and palliative care system. (Gesundheit Österreich, 2012) The manual covers three processes of: 1) from first contact to start of care, 2) care, and 3) bereavement support.

Volunteer training

Hospice Austria has three nationwide curricula for hospice and palliative care volunteers which are implemented in all nine federal states:

- Basic training (80 hours plus 40 hours practice)
- Hospice and palliative care for children and young people (an additional 40 hours and 40 hours practice)
- Bereavement support (an additional 80 hours for volunteers with basic training or 110 hours for volunteers without)

Volunteers must undertake training before they are allowed to work. This national approach enables qualified volunteers to work all over Austria. This applies to all volunteers involved in direct patient and family care. If volunteers are working in an office this training is not compulsory, but is recommended.

The main aim of the curriculum is to convey a certain mindset. The appropriate attitude is a volunteer's main instrument of care. It is the person herself/himself that is very important. A hospice volunteer's care is mainly characterized by the ability of staying present and simply being there as a companion, also by coping with feelings of helplessness and other strong emotions. Such a care requires a certain reticence from volunteers, an ability to cope with powerlessness, and an appreciation of differences. Therefore, learning from one's own experiences, self-reflection, and communication skills are woven throughout the training. Self-awareness is a key part of all learning.

The educational principles of learning are: 1. an open process with strong links to practice, 2. small groups, 3. learning by doing, and 4. learning by example. These principles are applied to the four fields of training content: a. biography, b. communication, c. information, and d. spirituality, with following main topics:

a. Field of biography

This area includes self-development, self-awareness, self-reflection, reflecting on one's own biography, and the role of volunteer care.

b. Field of communication

The field of communication comprises communication skills, social systems, group dynamics, conflict management, an understanding of the different levels of verbal and non-verbal communication; communication with frail people and people suffering from dementia.

c. Field of information

This third area covers graded hospice and palliative care institutions in Austria; basic medical and nursing knowledge in relevant palliative care topics (such as pain control, symptom control, eating, drinking,); basic ethical and legal knowledge in relevant topics (including living will, power of attorney, hospice leave); bereavement, dementia, and funerals.

d. Field of spirituality

This fourth part of training includes rites and rituals of dying and grief in the main religions; personal and general spiritual and religious needs; resources; attitude and values; spiritual care; the search for meaning; respect for other religions, world views, afterlife convictions.

All prospective hospice volunteers in Austria have to complete an application stating why they want to become a volunteer and what motivates them to do this.

Until the end of 2016 Hospice Austria chaired the National Forum on Bereavement Support (Bundesarbeitsgemeinschaft Trauerbegleitung, 2014) which developed an Austrian curriculum for bereavement support (Bundesarbeitsgemeinschaft Trauerbegleitung, 2014). As outlined earlier, there are two ways to qualify in this area, trained hospice volunteers can add the bereavement support qualification of 80 hours or a bereavement support qualification may be undertaken without a prior hospice volunteer qualification comprising 110 hours.

In order to start hospice and palliative care voluntary work for children, teenagers, and young adults, Hospice Austria developed a special curriculum which was issued in 2013. It is an advanced training for volunteers who have already worked with adults (Hospiz Österreich, 2013). By the end of 2015 Austria had 138 volunteers (82 of them in direct patient and family care) working in pediatric palliative care and eight new volunteer hospice teams for children and young people have started all around Austria.

The specific contribution that volunteers make is probably similar almost everywhere: having time, 'being there' sitting and listening, talking about life, awaking memories, taking a walk, or offering transport. Volunteers bring the normality of daily life to the patients and support their families and loved ones. In nursing homes they also carry out activities such as music, seat dancing, or reading to residents. Volunteers are also involved as board trustees, planning and organizing charity events, fundraising, and recruiting new people for hospice work.

Adequate financing is essential for voluntary hospice work. In Austria there is public funding for hospice teams, but it varies in all nine federal states. As a result, the availability of hospice services depends on the federal state where it is organized. This creates a significant need for private funding and fundraising in some parts of Austria.

In 2007 Hospice Austria started a partnership with the Austrian Savings Bank Group focusing on supporting the work of hospice volunteers. In most of the federal states there are projects where hospice teams are supported by local branches of the Austrian Savings Bank Group, Erste Bank, or the ERSTE Foundation. The support covers a wide range from financial support to providing an office and basic infrastructure or support in public relations and event management. In order to empower hospice work and the qualification of volunteers most of the financial resources received in this partnership are used for training, supervision, and team coordination.

Why and how volunteering in this field is changing

Demographic changes

During the last 20 years the hospice movement in Austria has gained strength, has become more confident, and continues to grow. Austrians nowadays have more information about what hospice and palliative care volunteers do and how they can help during the difficult time at the end of life. Also, due to demographic changes in society where more people reach old age, frailty and dementia increase and the baby boomer generation is approaching their 60s, coupled with the inclusion of non-cancer patient groups as recipients of hospice and palliative care; the need for this care is growing. Subsequently, there is a need to recruit and retain more volunteers.

New volunteers

On the other hand, volunteers have less time available and they volunteer less often and for shorter periods of time with more interest in project work. This presents a great challenge for organizations. Volunteers' motivation has changed too: in the past most people just wanted to help, nowadays so called 'new volunteers' also want to develop themselves personally and want to promote their professional career by volunteering. There are also more young volunteers, which is good for the age structure of voluntary hospice teams.

New target groups

Elderly people with dementia are becoming a new target group of hospice and palliative care: they bring new kinds of challenges and new requirements, including the need for training programmes.

Hospice and palliative care for children, teenagers, and young adults with life-limiting conditions has become a new and very challenging area of work. Tasks to be accomplished and questions arising differ from those already known from the adult sector. This requires new ways of thinking and creative solutions for the difficult situations these families are facing.

Bereavement is also a new growing area for hospice and palliative care volunteering with a need for specific training and new kinds of structures.

More complexity

The teams tell us that the complexity of the situation they encounter with patients and their families has increased and this calls for more and better qualifications. The family structures are more complex and people live longer with multi morbidities. There are many more patients with dementia and more people live alone. So, for example, some volunteers undertake further training, which helps them to empower patients with dementia.

Health and social care system

There are positive political processes and a high media interest with regards to hospice and palliative care in Austria.

Hospice and palliative care volunteers have become part of the Austrian health and social care system. The new challenges are now how to deal with more structure and less freedom and with growing administrative requirements through partial public funding. A challenge here is also keeping up the 'hospice spirit' in the health care system.

Factors that contribute to success

There are a number of elements that contribute to the success of hospice and palliative care volunteering.

Volunteer management and training

Proper management and coordination helps hospice and palliative care volunteering to reach its full potential and quality. Careful recruitment, selection, basic and ongoing training, supervision, and support are needed to ensure the quality of the volunteers' work. In this unique field of care, we need people with the right skills, values, and attitudes, and of course warm hearts. For hospice and palliative care volunteers this work means spending their time and using their talents in a meaningful way gaining personal growth and new experiences. If an organization can set the stage for making volunteering such an experience it will be successful in attracting and retaining volunteers.

An added factor that contributes to success is the person who coordinates the volunteer team, who is someone to whom volunteers can turn and is a valuable source of support.

Training, as outlined earlier in the chapter, also contributes significantly to success.

Standards and guidelines

In Austria the nationwide standards for volunteers and their managers set up by Hospice Austria are well known, implemented, and established across the whole country (Hospiz Österreich, 2002, 2008, 2011, 2013). Hospice Austria's annual data survey covers all hospice teams with many different aspects and information. This provides a good insight into volunteering and the development during the last ten years.

A factor of success at this level is to find the right balance between focus on standards and organization/management with the freedom of volunteering.

Proper funding

Proper funding is essential in order to be able to manage the voluntary teams effectively. Partnerships with Savings Bank Group, Erste Bank, and the ERSTE Foundation since 2007 have made it possible to ensure voluntary hospice work at a national level, federal state level, and local level. Without this support it would not have been possible to organize national or international symposia for volunteers. At the federal state and local level supervision and training could not have been developed so effectively. Additionally in Vienna there would be no paid coordinators without the financial support from ERSTE Foundation.

Cooperation between volunteers and paid staff

To be seen as equals is crucial when it comes to successful cooperation between volunteers and paid staff. Professional caregivers need to know what volunteer caregivers do and don't do and vice versa. Volunteers do not replace paid staff but have their own specific tasks. Hospice and palliative care volunteering can never be intended to replace professional palliative care. Professional care will always be needed in addition to the care provided by informal caregivers; family carers, and volunteers.

Culture and networking

The more we can integrate the 'hospice approach' in our society, e.g. schools and communities, the more volunteering can flourish. The more hospice and palliative care volunteering is seen as an expression of human values like solidarity and community caring, the more volunteering becomes an integral part of our society.

It is important to have good networking and cooperation with other hospice and palliative care and care organizations in order to offer the best care to the patient and his/her family. Cooperation can replace competition and it is much more motivating, enableing people to work together. In this way knowledge and information can be shared.

Appreciation

Volunteers' perspectives and opinions are heard and appreciated: volunteers as 'critical outsiders', but working in the hospice and palliative service are an important resource for the organization. Volunteers have a different perspective on the organization's strengths and weaknesses. They can offer valuable feedback to the professionals and to the organization on the way patients and their family/loved ones experience the care given and can therefore help to improve the quality of care.

Conclusion

There are many volunteers and volunteer coordinators all over Austria, who are working with great attitudes, warm hearts, and enthusiasm for hospice work. Volunteering has always been one of the core working areas of Hospice Austria.

In Austria hospice and palliative care volunteers are trained and prepared well for their unique task accompanying seriously ill and dying patients, their families, and loved ones. The volunteer hospice teams are well organized and managed and they work in close cooperation with other hospice and palliative care institutions. What is needed in Austria is more research yielding additional information in order to be well prepared for the changes that are necessary for volunteering to flourish in the future.

Co-chairing the EAPC Task Force on Volunteering in Hospice and Palliative Care gives great insight into other European countries. Being connected and learning from one another is the first step in meeting future challenges successfully!

References

Radbruch L., Payne S. et al. (2009) White Paper on standards and norms for hospice and palliative care in Europe: part 1.*European Journal of Palliative Care.* **16**(6) 278–89.

Parliamentary Commission of Enquiry (2014) Compare § 98. Available from: https://www.parlament.gv.at/ZUSD/RECHT/GOG-NR_DT-ENG-Taschenbuch_Volume1.pdf and https://www.parlament.gv.at/PAKT/VHG/XXV/I/I_00491/index.shtml

Gesundheit Österreich (Hg.) (2014) *Abgestufte Hospiz- und Palliativversorgung für Erwachsene* (Aktualisierung 2014) (Graded System for Hospice and Palliative Care Updated Version, 2014). Available from: http://www.bmgf.gv.at/cms/home/attachments/3/6/7/CH1071/CMS1103710970340/broschuere_hospiz-_und_palliativversorgung_1_12_2014.pdf

Gesundheit Österreich (Hg) (2012) *Prozesshandbuch Hospiz- und Palliativeinrichtungen* (Handbook for quality of processes). Available from: http://www.bmgf.gv.at/cms/home/attachments/3/6/7/CH1071/CMS1103710970340/prozesshandbuch_hospiz-_und_palliativeinrichtungen_02-11-2012.pdf

Nemeth, C., Pochobradsky, E. (2013) Hospiz- und Palliativversorgung für Kinder, Jugendliche und junge Erwachsene (Graded System for Hospice and Palliative Care for children and young adults). Available from: http://www.bmgf.gv.at/cms/home/attachments/3/6/7/CH1071/CMS1103710970340/hospiz-_und_palliativversorgung_fuer_kinder,_jugendliche_und_junge_erwachsene,_expertenkonzept_(2013).pdf

Hospiz Österreich (2002) *Standards für Österreich—Mindestanforderungen für die Einsatzkoordination im Mobilen Hospiz/Palliativdienst* (Standards for coordination of hospice teams). Available from: www.hospiz.at

Hospiz Österreich (2008) *Standards für ehrenamtlich tätige HospizbegleiterInnen* (Standards for hospice volunteers). Available from: www.hospiz.at

Hospiz Österreich (2011) *Curriculum für die Befähigungskurse ehrenamtlicher HospizbegleiterInnen* (Curriculum for volunteer training, updated version). Available from: www.hospiz.at

Hospiz Österreich (2013) *Curriculum zum Aufbaukurs zur ehrenamtlichen Hospizbegleitung von Kindern, Jugendlichen und jungen Erwachsenen* (Curriculum for hospice voluntary work for children, teenagers and young adults). Available from: www.hospiz.at

Bundesarbeitsgemeinschaft Trauerbegleitung (Hg) (2014) *Befähigung zur Trauerbegleiterin/zum Trauerbegleiter nach den Richtlinien der Bundesarbeitsgemeinschaft Trauerbegleitung* (Curriculum for bereavement support). Available from: http://www.trauerbegleiten.at/download/Curricula_BAG_Trauerbegleitung_lv.pdf

Chapter 5

Volunteering in hospice and palliative care in The Netherlands

Anne Goossensen and Jos Somsen

Introduction

The hospice and palliative care (HPC) movement in The Netherlands started out as a non-medical volunteer movement. The first palliative care organization in The Netherlands, founded in 1980, was a volunteer home care service aimed at enabling the terminally ill to die at home. Since the 1980s volunteering has developed rapidly in the home situation and from 1988 in hospices in The Netherlands. Now, in 2016, annually more than 11,000 volunteers provide different kinds of support at homes, and in hospices, and to a lesser extent in nursing homes. An umbrella organization (VPTZ Nederland) with around 200 member organizations develops policy, education, consultation for management and boards, and advocacy at a national level. Box 5.1 shows additional facts and figures from the Dutch umbrella organization VPTZ.

In this chapter we present the history of HPC volunteering in The Netherlands, we consider some figures and describe the structure of the organizations. Legislative and political influences are also discussed as well as approaches to management and training. Furthermore, we describe why and how volunteering in this field is changing and the factors that contribute to success. We conclude by describing some challenges for the future.

Brief history of palliative care volunteering in The Netherlands

Volunteer home care teams

The story of hospice and palliative care volunteering in The Netherlands started in 1971, with a young couple, Mr. and Mrs. Vriel (Slager, 2012). A few days after their first son was born, Mrs. Vriel was told that her husband was very ill. He was diagnosed with Hodgkin's disease at an advanced stage. The physician told Mrs Vriel her husband would have only a few months to live. The couple tried to cope

Box 5.1 Facts and figures for VPTZ Netherlands 2015

FACTS VPTZ Nederland (Dutch umbrella organization) 2015

- VPTZ Member organizations: 197 (incl. 114 hospices, with an average of five beds)
- Clients supported by volunteers: 11,199
- Volunteers: 10,893
- Average hrs/client: 130 (home: 37, hospice: 213)
- Average duration of support: 24 days
- Total hrs volunteers/year: 1,336,571 hours
- 88 per cent of hours in care-focussed roles
- 516 (mostly paid) volunteer coordinators
- National Curriculum for volunteers, coordinators and board members
- Volunteer involvement in 12 per cent of non-acute deaths at national level (in 2012)
- Funding of hospices by governments (62 per cent), clients (14 per cent) and fundraising (24 per cent)

Reproduced courtesy VPTZ Nederland. Source: data from VPTZ Nederland. *Registratierapportage 2015 [Registration report 2015].* VPTZ Nederland, Amersfoort, The Netherlands, Copyright © 2016 VPTZ Nederland.

with this situation. Neither in their social network, nor among their physicians, was support found for them in trying to live with an incurable disease. It was not only a lack of understanding, it also seemed impossible to address the topic in conversations. The topic was neglected, a taboo. Mrs. Vriel, who was studying nursing, organized fellow nursing students to help her care for Mr. Vriel. In this way they managed to keep him at home until his death, five years later: a unique situation for The Netherlands.

After two years the couple got in touch with a newspaper. A journalist interviewed them on a regular basis and became closely involved with the couple. He wrote 40 articles about their situation which were subsequently published as a book (Sinner, 1976). At that time, more care became available for palliative patients enabling them to stay at home longer.

To facilitate staying at home until the end Mrs. Vriel organized a group for people in similar situations. This evolved into an organization that enabled people to die at home. Volunteers helped patients with going to the toilet, dressing, or preparing food. They only assisted, and did not take over responsibilities. In 1980, four years after her husband's death, Mrs. Vriel and others started the Leendert Vriel foundation aiming to assist terminal patients to die at home with the assistance of volunteers. The foundation received national and international attention resulting in familiar initiatives all over the country. In 1984 these initiatives came together in a foundation called Volunteers Terminal Care (VTZ), with a national office that supported new initiatives and provided training and advocacy at a national level.

Almost-like-home-houses

Soon after these first initiatives several Dutch pioneers got in touch with the development of hospices in Great Britain (Bruntink, 2002). A general practitioner (GP), named Pieter Sluis, initiated a Kübler-Ross Foundation in The Netherlands. It aimed at spreading ideas about conscious dying and bereavement. Sluis visited St Christopher's hospice in London, and although he was sympathetic towards the initiative, he felt it was too much of an institution. He envisioned a setting on a much smaller scale embedded in the local community and run by volunteers. In 1986 his group opened the first 'almost-like-home-house', a uniquely Dutch concept of a hospice: a house run by volunteers, with volunteers in care-focused roles at the core of the organization, where patients could spend the last stage of their lives, if that was not possible in the home situation. Many 'almost-like-home-houses' (typically with around four beds) were founded all over the country. Similar to home situations most of the care in the almost-like-home-houses is provided by informal caregivers, i.e. family carers and trained volunteers. Professional carers (nurses, doctors, therapists) come in to provide the professional care as needed. In most of the 'almost-like-home-houses' there is 24/7 availability, but not the 24/7 presence of trained nurses. The continuity of care is assured by the presence of volunteers during the day and evenings (although the night care is often provided primarily by a nurse). Sluis also founded the Dutch Hospice Movement in 1996, the first umbrella organization for hospices that combined with the foundation Volunteers Terminal Care to form VPTZ Nederland in 2005.

High-care hospices

In 1987, almost at the same time as the birth of a first almost-like-home-house, a priest, Rob van Hellenberg Hubar started another foundation. This Elckerlijck Foundation promoted consciousness around dying and living. This organization supported the hospice thought by understanding dying as a process of inner growth. Both the Kübler-Ross and Elckerlijck Foundations promoted the understanding of dying not as the ultimate failing of medicine, but as a normal

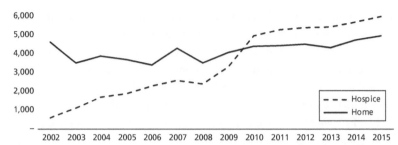

Figure 5.1 Number of clients supported by volunteers in hospices and at home

Reproduced courtesy VPTZ Nederland. Source: data from VPTZ Nederland. *Registratierapportage 2014 [Registration report 2014]*. VPTZ Nederland, Amersfoort, The Netherlands, Copyright © 2016 VPTZ.

phase of life. In 1994 this resulted in another type of hospice, founded together with the Salvation Army, and modelled after the English hospices (although much smaller in scale), with a multi-disciplinary team of care professionals, but also a large group of volunteers. Around the same time, other so-called high-care hospices (with multidisciplinary care teams) from other backgrounds started, with typically around seven beds, and also the significant involvement of volunteers, both in care-focused and more facilitative roles. The high-care hospices started their own umbrella organization, the Association of Hospice Care The Netherlands. Currently VPTZ Nederland and the Association are working towards closer collaboration.

Nowadays VPTZ Nederland has around 200 member organizations. Together these member organizations run 87 almost-like-home-houses, 18 high-care hospices and nine palliative care units (units in nursing homes that also have significant involvement of volunteers) and 135 volunteer home-care teams. In 2015 10,893 volunteers were working in these organizations. In 2012 VPTZ volunteers were involved in the care of 12 per cent of non-acute deaths. In 2015, 53 per cent of the people supported by volunteers stayed in a hospice, 44 per cent in their own homes and 2 per cent in other settings (mostly nursing homes). In the home situation around one third of the volunteer hours took place during the night (Figure 5.1).

Legislative and political influences

While the roots of volunteering in hospices and in the home situation in The Netherlands lie in the 1980s, in the 1990s the field of palliative care became fully recognized by the Ministry of Health, being strongly supported by Minister Els Borst, who also played an important role in legalizing euthanasia. The first subsidy regulations were established in the mid 1990s, providing the hospice and palliative care (HPC) volunteering organizations with some basic financial support. Although this was of great help to the HPC volunteering organizations, the amount of subsidies available also varied greatly across the nation.

In 2007 the current state subsidy regulations were established, providing all the HPC volunteer organizations in The Netherlands with a steady flow of basic finances for housing and coordination, based on the amount of clients supported in a certain period, either at their home or in a hospice. These state subsidies constitute, on average, 59 per cent of the volunteer organizations' finances. Other money is raised by the organizations themselves through local fundraising activities, patients' contributions, and private project funding. By granting these subsidies the state recognizes the importance of this work and the need for good volunteer management, by reimbursing part of the local organizations' costs for management and coordination, and the hospices' costs for housing. This state subsidy regulation especially for HPC volunteering is quite unique for The Netherlands, since all other subsidies for local volunteering organizations are provided by local government, and a recent change in the state subsidy regulations for volunteering in HPC has made it possible to also use the subsidy for supporting people in care and nursing homes. Because in 2012 roughly one third (35 per cent) of the non-acute deaths occurred in care and nursing homes, we expect a substantial rise in the requests for our volunteers' support in the near future. Figure 5.2 shows data for the place of death in 2012 (VPTZ Nederland, 2014). The improvement of palliative care is regarded as a high priority by most of The Netherlands' politicians and by the government. This has resulted in a five-year state funded National Programme for Palliative Care, combining the development of practice, research, and education. One focus of the programme is the collaboration of professional carers with family

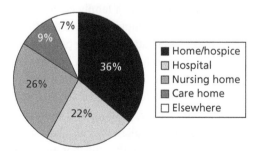

Figure 5.2 Place of non-acute deaths in 2012

Reproduced courtesy VPTZ Nederland. Source: data from VPTZ Nederland. *Registratierapportage 2014 [Registration report 2014]*. VPTZ Nederland, Amersfoort, The Netherlands, Copyright © 2015 VPTZ.

carers and HPC volunteers. Another influential political development is the end of the welfare state in The Netherlands. Since health care costs were becoming too high, government policy looked for possibilities to cut the costs of professional care. By the introduction of the 'participation community' concept much more care is expected from close ones (family, neighbours, friends) and from volunteers within the local communities. Because the relatives are expected to take up more care, we expect they will also need more support from volunteers to be able to cope with the situation. The government promotes good collaboration between professional and informal forms of care. HPC volunteering in The Netherlands has a lot of experience in closely collaborating with family carers and professional carers and can therefore be a model for this kind of collaboration, also for other fields of care.

Approaches to management and training

Management of volunteering

The management models of volunteering vary with the different care settings. One form of hospice—the almost-like-home-houses—and the volunteer home care services are mostly volunteer run organizations. The community volunteers (both in care-focused and in more facilitative roles) are supervised by the coordinators of their volunteer organization. These (mostly paid) coordinators are not necessarily health care professionals, and when they are, they do not work within their discipline. This is because these volunteer-led organizations are not officially health care organizations. The clients of these volunteer services receive professional care (doctors, nurses, other therapists) from the general health care system, both at home and in the almost-like-home-houses. The volunteers in these organizations work together with family carers and professionals on the basis of equality, each giving care from within their own role and speciality. The care of family carers is based on their relationship to the dying person. The volunteers add to this from within their role of 'being there' for the client and relatives, and the professional carers add skills and knowledge from their own professional discipline and expertise.

The position of the coordinators is central within these organizations. They work directly under the board (volunteers themselves) and lead the group of volunteers. Apart from coordinating, training, and supervising the volunteers and their work with patients and families, they also have a major role in policy making, public relations, organizing the collaboration between volunteers and professional and family carers, admitting patients to the service, and (in hospices) running the house. They play a key role as a liaison between the board and the volunteer team. They may run into time problems and perform part of their tasks in their own time. Also the quality of the board may vary, which may sometimes put the coordinator in a difficult position in between volunteers and a voluntary board. This can risk overburdening the coordinator.

There are two other forms of hospice where volunteers may play a significant role, called high-care hospices and palliative units within care or nursing homes. These are essentially health care organizations, with nurses and other professionals on their payroll. They may have bigger or smaller groups of HPC volunteers, in care-giving roles and in facilitative roles. In these organizations the volunteers tend to have less of an independent role. There is usually a volunteer coordinator, but the care-focused volunteers mostly work under the supervision of a nurse. Also, the role of the coordinator is more restricted, for instance they have less responsibility in running the house, admitting patients to the service, etc. HPC volunteers from the volunteer home services that work in nursing homes are supervised by their own organization's coordinator, but of course within the nursing home, they collaborate closely with the paid staff.

Education

Accurate and careful recruitment, selection, initial and continuous training, reflection, and supervision are of crucial importance in all Dutch settings where volunteers work; especially those who work in care-related roles who need to have at least the following qualities:

- Communication skills (ability to listen without judgement, attune to the client's needs, etc.)
- Having processed their own bereavement experiences enough to be able to be there for someone else
- Ability to reflect upon and learn from one's own experiences
- Clarity about one's role and position as a HPC volunteer (in relation to family carers and professional carers)
- Understanding and respecting differences in personal values and being able to act towards others accordingly

Providing good quality of care by volunteers requires clear policy and good management and coordination of the volunteers' efforts.

After the initial interview, suitable candidates attend seven training sessions, organized by the local volunteer organization and led by a coordinator who has been trained for this purpose or a professional trainer. VPTZ Nederland developed a national curriculum for this course, supported by e-learning. The training covers topics like the position of volunteers within HPC and within the organization, bereavement, values around death and dying, practical care, hygiene, and safety. The training is also part of the selection process. After this initial training both the candidate and the volunteer coordinator decide whether they want to continue the collaboration. The volunteer then starts his or her work as a volunteer, receiving supervision from the coordinator, regular evaluation or training sessions within the organization, and sometimes also collegial consultation groups with other volunteers. In these meetings horizontal reflection takes place between volunteers based on a difficult situation that one of them has experienced.

In the training programmes the focus is on learning by reflection and learning from peers. Much of the training is aimed at reflecting on actual experiences, where 'being there' posed difficulties or dilemmas. Volunteers reflect on questions like: What was at stake for me in this situation? Could I see or sense the other person's need? Did I have inner space to be open to the other person? Was there a good connection between the other person and me?

Apart from this training and supervision within local organizations, VPTZ Nederland also provides an extended (voluntary) national training programme for volunteers, directors/managers/coordinators and board members, combining e-learning with face-to-face learning in groups (blended learning). In 2015, 1500 volunteers and 225 coordinators and board members were trained within the national training programme. This programme is partly financed by the Dutch state. Topics also include diversity, dementia, basic knowledge about terminal illnesses, ethics, management, and leadership. For board members VPTZ Nederland organizes masterclasses to facilitate sharing both expert knowledge and actual experiences.

Why and how volunteering in this field is changing

Developments in the request for HPC volunteering

A substantial rise in the request for HPC volunteering is expected within the next years. Earlier in this chapter we have already mentioned the new subsidy regulations that support HPC volunteering within nursing and care homes. Gains are to be expected for the frail elderly who have very few (or no) family or friends left and can greatly benefit from the company and support of specialized volunteers in their last stage of life along with their remaining families. Large organizations of elderly people have started to promote volunteers as important enablers of dignified dying at home.

Other developments that will lead to a rise in demand for HPC volunteers include:

◆ The expected rise of non-acute deaths from 81,000 in 2012 to 100,000 in 2020

◆ The government policy aimed at people staying home as long as possible and also to die at home and less in hospitals, nursing homes or care homes

- The government policy to provide less professional care and expect more from family care and volunteers
- The diminishing amount of family care available, due to smaller families (fewer children to take care of their parents), separations, more people that live on their own, people working longer into old age, and more women in the workforce that do not have a lot of time left to take care of family members (or work as a volunteer).

Developments in the field of volunteering

Although until now no great difficulties have been reported in finding enough HPC volunteers, this is expected to become a greater challenge in the near future. Apart from the previously mentioned challenges around the amount of time left for volunteering (due to working longer into old age, more women in the labour force, more time needed for family care), the field of volunteering in general is changing in more and different ways.

One of the developments is that people tend to commit less to an organization and more to a certain project or time-limited task within their own discipline. For instance a public relations (PR) consultant may be happy to write a PR plan for the organization, or a construction worker may be willing to volunteer his/her time and skills to a hospice building project. Volunteers that do commit to the organization for a longer period of time may have less time available during the week then in earlier days, because they have other important things they want to devote their time to. These developments may be challenging for the organizations to accommodate. On the other hand, Dutch volunteers tend to value personal development more than they used to, and want to participate more in decision making. To meet these needs Dutch HPC volunteer organizations' focus on training and personal feedback and development has the potential of tapping into those needs and wishes very effectively.

One aspect of the political developments in health care policy is the fact that volunteering receives a lot of positive attention and tends to get valued more explicitly. Also, professional carers and insurance companies look much more to volunteer organizations as valuable partners to collaborate with, for the sake of the patient and of course for the sake of the efficient use of scarce money and resources. The challenging side of this is that not everybody understands that cutting down on professional care without making investments in volunteering is not going to work, and that volunteers can never be seen as a replacement of paid care workers. Also the risk exists that volunteers and their organizations are asked to do things they are not equipped or suited to do, like medical or nursing tasks, when there are not enough professionals to take on this work. It also happens that patients are referred to (volunteer-led or high-care) hospices, not because this is the best place for them to be, but because the referring professional can't find a suitable place in a nursing home for them to be cared for.

Another challenge that the Dutch volunteer organizations are facing is the growing complexity of the patients' problems. For instance, the fact that people with dementia will stay in their own homes for much longer means that the volunteers are faced with problems associated with dementia (in the patient or the prime family carer) much more often. This calls for clear policy within the local organization around the tasks volunteers can and cannot do, and around the clients that can or cannot be served by the organization. Also, with shifting boundaries it is important to adequately guide and train the volunteers for the more complex tasks they will do, and make them confident in setting boundaries, knowing their own limitations, and referring patients to professional care when needed.

Moreover, another important development in The Netherlands is the building of closer connections between the volunteering organizations and the professional care organizations, especially within home care. This asks for attention at the level of organizations. For instance, GPs and community nurses have started to work together in palliative care teams, around a method including early recognition, advanced care planning, and ongoing education. There are about 100 of these teams now called Palliative Care in the Home situation (PaTz), and some of these teams include coordinators from HPC volunteering organizations (both hospice and home care volunteering organizations). This is a promising development that will greatly benefit the multidisciplinary and multi-dimensional care for people that die in their own home, and their relatives. Furthermore actions at micro level are necessary. A further clarification of the identity of volunteers resulting in clear criteria for success is needed.

Success factors

Factors that have greatly helped HPC volunteering to blossom in The Netherlands, based on observations that have been highlighted, include:

+ The clear positioning of HPC volunteering alongside family care and professional care, with its own non-medical role, with the core value of 'being there'
+ The unique Dutch hospice concepts of small-scale community-based 'almost-like-home-houses' (with volunteers at the core of the organization) and the relatively small-scale high-care hospices with considerable numbers of volunteers in care-focused and facilitative roles
+ The existence of strong community based volunteer home care teams and their increasingly close collaboration with professional home care teams

- The existence of a grass roots national umbrella organization, that organizes advocacy, education/training, consultation, and policy at a national level, specifically for HPC volunteering in hospices and home care organizations
- Strong support from the national government for palliative care in general and HPC volunteering in particular, characterized both by volunteering-friendly policies and regulations and substantial funding for the volunteering organizations
- The establishment of an Academic Chair dedicated to HPC volunteering in The Netherlands. This will contribute to the positioning of HPC volunteering and generate knowledge about the identity, value, and quality of volunteering in The Netherlands and elsewhere

Identity: being there

The existence of strong local volunteer-based organizations is powerful in defining and positioning volunteering as a unique form of care alongside professional and family care. But because volunteers in the home situation are usually not part of multi-disciplinary teams within one organization, they may be easily overlooked by both professional carers and patients. They are not always seen and valued as an integral part of the chain of care necessary to provide good support and total care to the patient and their close ones. A clear description of their identity will contribute to success in several ways. At the European level, the Task Force Volunteering of the European Association for Palliative Care (EAPC) chose the concept of 'being there' as the essence of hospice and palliative care volunteering in care-focussed roles. Throughout all member organizations and countries this concept is communicated as the rationale for successful hospice and palliative care volunteering.

'Being there' means 'becoming who the other needs' including being emotionally or existentially available to be with what is at stake for the other. This 'being there' raises theoretical questions. Can it be considered a competence? A talent? A skill? Can it be learned and improved? Is selection possible based on performed quality of being there? To understand fully the potential of being there a connection with theories of presence can be made. This means that 'being there' cannot simply be understood as 'just' being there in the sense of physical presence. Being there in line with presence theories requires more in the sense of becoming totally open to receive the smallest signal from the other, from a position of wanting to understand and meet the other. Theories on presence seem to stem from at least two different disciplinary backgrounds: nursing sciences and theology.

Far more descriptions were found in the literature on nursing. Being there understood from these insights has a dimension of being sensitive and receptive to the otherness of the other. It is more than being totally in the here and the now as described by mindfulness, although this will surely help to reach the sensitive searching for the other.

Several descriptions understand presence as more than a characteristic of the attitude of a carer but understand it as a relational quality. Covington (2005) calls it 'a way of being and relating' and Anderson (2007) writes about 'being in an authentic relationship'. Doona (1997) describes nursing presence as an 'intersubjective encounter in which the nurse decides to spend herself on the patients' behalf'. Hines (1992) notes that the encounter should be valued and that connectedness should be reached. This shines light on results of being there in the present: it nurtures good connections and relationships in palliative care.

To summarize the understanding of being there from a nursing presence perspective means to be there fully for the other, with an open attention and to listen in a way that allows receiving, from an attitude that wants to be with the other, aiming for reciprocity and trying to spend oneself on what is perceived to be important. As Zerwekh (1997) writes: 'be there, meet them where they are at.'

What do volunteers say about their experiences of 'being there'? From a qualitative research study based on 100 letters from volunteers in palliative care (Goossensen and Sakkers, 2014) a volunteer expresses:

> Being there for our guests and their families is a recurring aspect wherein one can unfold. Thanks to the experience with the guests one learns again and again how to act or to act not. We are in the background and we observe. Say something or remain silent. We accompany people to the other side at their pace and in their manner of doing. Every human is unique, every dying is unique and we are privileged to be present there. The special thing is that at the moment of death every human returns to his own I. With all of his or her life lessons. We as volunteers can take care or at least try to make that last road as comfortable as possible. (Female volunteer, age 55; Goossensen and Sakkers, 2014)

'Being there' then proves to become a layered and nuanced term. It involves much more than only physical presence. It contains withholding yourself, emptying, being silent, offering space, sensitive tuning, and being attentive. Based on this a volunteer 'reads' who the other person is, what the situation is, and what might be his or her response. Another Dutch volunteer writes in a letter project:

> The term 'Being there' is much more comprehensive than I had thought. Sometimes you just have a talk with someone. Sometime you only have to be present and you read a book half way through. On another occasion someone pours out immediately upon your entering the room. At the first acquaintance! That I find so special. With other

people it is not so clear what they expect from me. I then try to 'read' them. What would they prefer? Do they want to talk or rather not? And if they do not wish to talk: how do I see that I remain approachable in case they do want to ask anything. (Female volunteer, age 56; Goossensen and Sakkers, 2014)

Volunteers express satisfaction, gratefulness, and see benefits for themselves as well. They report that they grow, due to the work in the hospices or with people at the end of life at their homes. A third Dutch volunteer writes:

What this work brought me personally is insights into who I am myself. It enriched me enormously as a human and it still deepens the way I live. It encouraged me to study as a 'giving meaning therapist'. What I learn there, I have been able to put into practice within the hospice. It also encourages me to a more intense life. What really values for me, what I am in need of. Also because of this I started to change things, lay off things so that others can profit from these, shut down things that are not of value anymore. Hectic life in society is not welcome to me anymore. (Female volunteer, age 45; Goossensen and Sakkers, 2014)

Value of volunteering

For volunteers both quality assessment and transparency on results of volunteering are needed more and more in order to count and be recognized in the complex care field. Only mentioning positive experiences is not enough anymore. How can we best express the value of the volunteers' effort? In The Netherlands only the satisfaction data of family members have been gathered in a pilot. In the international literature results suggested that patients who have the support of volunteers live longer (Herbst-Damm and Kulik, 2005), and that care is more often graded as excellent the more hours volunteers have been involved (Block et al., 2010). In The Netherlands we are now evaluating dignity as an outcome measure of volunteering.

Challenges for the future

There are many challenges for the future. It would be helpful to undertake further theoretical and empirical exploration and understanding of 'being there'. This could have value for the selection, education, and quality assessments for hospice and palliative care volunteering (Goossensen, 2016). For instance, researchers who consider the possibilities for a quality system based on this concept could try to identify research instruments that evaluate quality of 'being there'.

In determining the quality of volunteering, finding sufficient outcome indicators for successful volunteer caring, while at the same time not considering volunteering as an intervention is a theoretical challenge. It is possible that considering the 'dignity' of patients may be a promising concept.

Finally, more and more volunteers appear to have added value for palliative care in elderly care homes. More knowledge about what is required to make this successful is needed, including the necessary factors for effective collaboration between professional and volunteer carers.

Acknowledgements

Text extracts from Goossensen A. and Sakkers M. *'Daar doe ik het voor.'* *Ervaringen van vrijwilligers in de palliatieve zorg* ['That's what's in it for me.' Volunteers' experiences in palliative care]. VPTZ Nederland, Amersfoort, The Netherlands, Copyright © 2014 The authors. Reproduced courtesy VPTZ Nederland.

References

Andersson, B., and Ohlén, J. (2005) Being a hospice volunteer. *Palliat Med* **19**: 602–9.

Anderson J.H. (2007) The Impact of Using Nursing Presence in a Community Heart Failure Program. *Journal of Cardiovascular Nursing* **22**(2): 89–94.

Block, E.M., Casarett, D.J., Spence, C. et al. (2010) Got volunteers? Association of hospice use of volunteers with bereaved family members' overall rating of the quality of end-of-life care. *J Pain Symptom Manage* **39**(3): 502–6.

Bruntink, R. (2002) *Een goede plek om te sterven. Palliatieve zorg in Nederland. [A good place to die. Palliative care in The Netherlands.]* Zutphen: Uitgeverij Plataan.

Covington H. (2005) Caring presence: providing a safe space for patients. Holist Nurs Pract **19**(4):169–172.

Doona, M.E., Haggerty, L.A., and Chase, S.K. (1997). Nursing Presence: An Existential Exploration of the Concept. *Scholarly Inquiry for Nursing Practice* **11**(1): 3–16.

Goossensen, A. (2016) *Naar de poëtica van de ander. De waarde van vrijwilligers in de palliatieve zorg.* [Towards the poetics of the other. The value of volunteers in palliative care.] Oratie. University of Humanistic Studies, Utrecht [Inaugural adress].

Goossensen, A. and Sakkers, M. (2014) 'Daar doe ik het voor.' Ervaringen van vrijwilligers in de palliatieve zorg. ['That's what's in it for me.' Volunteers' experiences in palliative care.] Uitgave: VPTZ Nederland.

Herbst-Damm, K.L. and Kulik, J.A. (2005) Volunteer support, marital status, and the survival times of terminally ill patients. *Health Psychol* **24**(2): 225–9.

Hines, D.R. (1992) Presence. Discovering the Artistry in Relating. *Journal of Holistic Nursing* **10**(4): 294–305.

VPTZ Nederland (2014) *Antenne nr. 123, maart 2014: 30 jaar VPTZ [30 years VPTZ].* Bunnik: VPTZ Nederland.

VPTZ Nederland (2016). *Registratierapportage 2015 [Registration report 2015].* Amersfoort: VPTZ Nederland.

VPTZ Nederland (2014). *VPTZ Trendrapport 2014 [VPTZ Trend report].* Bunnik: VPTZ Nederland.

Zerwekh J.V. (1997) The practice of presencing. *Semin Oncol Nurs* **13**(4): 260–2.

Chapter 6

Volunteering in hospice and palliative care in Germany

Michaela Hesse and Lukas Radbruch

Brief history

The history of the hospice movement in Germany started with a misunderstanding. In 1971 a film following a patient in London's St Christopher's Hospice called 'Only 16 days' was broadcast on German television. In this film the term 'Hospice' was translated as 'hospital for dying' (Sterbeklinik). This led to associations linking hospices with euthanasia and holocaust. Both Catholic and Protestant church authorities opposed hospice development, fearing that hospices could become ghettos for the dying. This discussion delayed the development of hospice and palliative care in Germany for more than ten years.

The initial hospice or palliative care initiatives and model projects started in the 1980s (Aulbert et al., 2012). The first inpatient service was established as a palliative care unit within the surgical department at the University of Cologne in 1983. The service formed after discussions about the need for palliative care in Germany between Heinz Pichlmaier, the head of the surgical department and Mildred Scheel, a physician herself and the wife of the German president at that time, when she required treatment for cancer. The hospital chaplain Helmut Zielinski had just returned from St Christopher's hospice in London, and had suggested something similar for the hospital. From the first unit starting as five beds in three rooms and a living room on the 17th floor of the hospital building, the dedicated staff, led by Ingeborg Jonen-Thielemann, soon did much to disseminate palliative care ideas and attitudes. Two more inpatient palliative care units opened in 1986 at the Malteser Hospital and the Janker Hospital, both in Bonn.

The first inpatient hospice was affiliated to the nursing home 'Haus Hörn' in Aachen in 1986 Here the initiative was driven by Paul Türks, one of the Catholic chaplains of the nursing home. This was soon followed by hospices in Recklinghausen ('Hospiz zum Heiligen Franziskus') and in Frankfurt ('Christopherus Haus') which both opened in 1987.

Since then there has been slow but steady progress for palliative medicine in Germany. In the last two decades there have been more inpatient units established so that by 2015, there were 286 palliative care units (those that are in hospitals) and 217 inpatient hospices providing an average of 30.5 palliative care beds and 27.31 hospice beds per million inhabitants (Melching, 2015). In addition, there were 241 specialized palliative home care teams registered in Germany in 2015, corresponding to 2.98 teams per million inhabitants. In contrast to other countries, in Germany the development of hospice care was not linked to the development of palliative care. Therefore inpatient hospices are nurse or volunteer-led and the provision of medical care is covered by general practitioners (GPs). Palliative care units are physician-led hospital inpatient units.

The provision of palliative care has reached a state of advanced integration in mainstream health care, as ranked in the atlas of palliative care (Worldwide Palliative Care Alliance, 2014). Germany was ranked seventh in a quality of death evaluation in 2015, with only UK, Ireland, and Belgium ranking higher in Europe (Economist Intelligence Unit, 2015). However, even with the excellent stage of development, palliative care or hospice interventions were only documented for 29.6 per cent of all dying patients in a large sickness funds survey, whereas a need for palliative care would be estimated for as many as 90 per cent of the dying. Only 3.5 per cent of the dying had received specialist palliative home care for a median duration of 24 days in the last year of life, but 12.2 per cent of these patients had accessed this specialist home care only in the last three days of life, something we would suggest is too late.

Looking at this history, we can see that the development of hospice care was not linked to that of palliative medicine in Germany. Hospice care developed as a civil society movement often led by engaged volunteers while the development of palliative medicine got started with a focus on specialized palliative care led by a few pioneer physicians. This separate development is still visible in the organizational structures, as a clear distinction between palliative care units and inpatient hospices has developed in Germany.

Volunteering in hospice care started in parallel with this professional development as a citizens' movement. This was motivated by an increasing feeling of unease with the denial of death and dying in modern society. It was felt that dying should no longer take place in isolation, secreted away in the bathrooms or storerooms of hospital wards. There was a strong feeling that society needed more awareness of the end-of-life and of how to support patients with a life-limiting disease and their caregivers to stay at home until the very end, to enable them to die in their familiar surroundings and with their loved ones at the bedside. So the history of volunteering started with Johann-Christoph

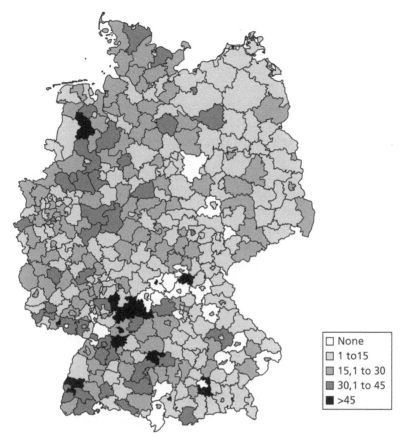

Figure 6.1 Volunteer services in Germany per million inhabitants, at district level
Reproduced with permission from Melching, H. *Palliativversorgung Modul 2: Strukturen und regionale Unterschiede in der Hospiz- und Palliativversorgung,* Bertelsmann Stiftung, Copright © 2015.
Source: data from Wegweiser Hospiz- und Palliativmedizin. www.wegweiser-hospiz-palliativmedizin.de

Student and his workgroup 'Zuhause sterben' (dying at home) in Hannover in 1984, and in the same year the taskforce 'Arbeitsgemeinschaft Sitzwachen' (bedside vigil) was established in Stuttgart. The 'St. Christopher Hospiz-Verein' (St. Christopher Hospice Association), the first non-government organization (NGO) in Germany to have the word hospice in its name, was established in 1985 in Munich, with the aim of establishing an inpatient hospice. The OMEGA association was founded in the same year, and Paul Becker, who had implemented palliative care in his general practice as one of the first physicians in Germany, founded the 'Internationale Gesellschaft für Sterbebegleitung und Lebenshilfe' (International Association for Care of the Dying and Counselling) in 1986. The

'Bundesarbeitsgemeinschaft Hospiz' (Federal Hospice Working Group) was established in 1992, the German Association for Palliative Medicine in 1995. A German hospice directory with addresses and services provided has been issued regularly since 1993 and is now available online (http://www.wegweiser-hospiz-palliativmedizin.de).

Palliative care and hospice volunteering today has become firmly established in Germany as an integral part of the care of severely ill and dying patients. In 2002 there were 102 hospices, 77 palliative care units and around 1,100 volunteer services. At that time approximately 45,000 voluntary workers accomplished 711,500 volunteer hours in out-patient care and 98,000 volunteer hours were provided in stationary hospice care (Deutscher Bundestag 15. Wahlperiode). In 2015 the hospice directory listed 1,370 volunteer services, including 117 volunteer services for children and adolescents, resulting in an average of 15.55 services per million inhabitants (Figure 6.1).

Having this dual history of physician-led and volunteer-led approach inevitably led to tensions between the services but these are being mitigated, though are still sometimes visible, with the ongoing development of palliative and hospice care. With palliative medicine as a medical (sub) specialty on one hand and volunteering as a citizens' movement on the other hand they are improving their collaboration in local and regional networks.

Legislative and political influences

The new hospice and palliative care law (HPG) clarified that health care has to include palliative care with an amendment in clause 27 of the 5th volume of the code of social law, introducing a general right to access palliative care in the German health care system. Palliative Care always includes involvement of volunteers. The HPG confirmed that and also introduced an obligation for nursing homes to collaborate with a volunteer service, requiring a formal cooperation agreement (Bundesgesetzblatt, 2015). The HPG was passed in December 2015, but even before this volunteers have been, and remain an essential part of the provision of hospice and palliative care in Germany, and this is shown in how volunteering has been represented in the legislation introduced during the last two decades. Specialized palliative home care teams (as regulated in clause 37b of the 5th volume of the code of social law) and inpatient hospices (clause 39a of the 5th volume of the code of social law) are obliged to collaborate with a volunteer service.

Volunteers are in most cases organized in volunteer services (Ambulante Hospizdienste, AHD) and coordinated by professional volunteer coordinators. Volunteers are trained and supervised by qualified coordinators of the service.

Coordinators have to have training in a health care profession or social work, training in palliative care, and have at least three years working experience in palliative or hospice care. Coordinator qualifications also have to include training in coordination (40 hours) and leadership skills (80 hours) to be eligible for reimbursement of costs by the sickness funds.

Volunteers are most often with patients in their home care setting, but they also accompany patients during hospital stays. Volunteers provide psychosocial support for patients and their families—independent of the setting—and are able to engage with patients and families on the same level, that is, without the hierarchical distance that can typify relations between health care professionals and patients. By providing this for patients they also add a patient-centred perspective to the multi-professional palliative care team that will include physicians, nurses, social workers, spiritual workers, psychologists, and therapists.

Volunteer services also offer bereavement services, mostly with low-level interventions such as bereavement cafés, but also with individual counselling and support. Many of the volunteers working in these services have had additorial training for bereavement support.

Costs of coordinator salaries, training costs, and some costs for materials are reimbursed by sickness funds (a form of medical insurance) and to claim this money an organization documents the number of patients accompanied by volunteers to the sickness funds. For example, if the volunteer service has 15 or more trained volunteers and a qualified coordinator staff costs may be reimbursed by the sickness funds. However, not all services receive reimbursement from the sickness funds. For example in 2014 the sickness funds reported that 841 volunteer services received reimbursement out of a total of 1,370. The other services either cover their expenses by charity fund raising, or are still in the process of establishing a volunteer support service.

The German health care system offers other options for hospice and palliative care, including specialist care in palliative care units and inpatient hospices, or with specialized teams providing palliative care at home or in nursing homes. Basic palliative care is delivered by home-care nursing services or by the general practitioners. In some federal states such as North Rhine-Westphalia nursing services may have special contracts for nursing palliative care. There are also a number of model projects using different approaches throughout Germany.

In contrast to other countries, there are fundamental differences in the scope of work of palliative care units and inpatient hospices in Germany. Admission to a palliative care unit is only possible if inpatient hospital treatment is indicated. Palliative care units are organized as hospital units and are funded from the sickness fund health insurance. Patients are admitted to treat symptoms or distress but the aim is always to discharge the patient to return home or to a hospice as soon as possible and the mean inpatient length of stay is less than two weeks. Overall approximately half of patients are discharged, whereas fewer than half are admitted in their terminal phase and stay in the unit until their death. Palliative care is a medical subspecialty in Germany, but many palliative care units are affiliated with other departments of the hospital, most frequently oncology.

Costs for treatment in the palliative care unit can follow two models: either reimbursement follows the German Diagnostics Related Groups (DRG) system, with a special code for complex palliative care (Zusatzentgelt komplexe Palliativversorgung auf einer Palliativstation ZE 145), or the unit is exempted from the DRG system and is paid with a flat fee per patient day. This flat fee is negotiated by each hospital with the sickness funds in the yearly budget negotiations (in North Rhine-Westphalia between 420 and 480 Euros per patient day).

Inpatient hospice care is for patients who are in the final phase of their disease, during the final weeks or months of life, and do not require inpatient hospital resources. They are staffed with nurses, and have few resources for medical, social, and spiritual care. Hospices do not have physicians on their staff, and medical care is usually provided by a GP.

Patients may be admitted to an inpatient hospice if they are unable to stay at home because there is no caregiver or because care needs are too big, but are not requiring inpatient hospital care. Inpatient hospices are reimbursed with a flat fee per day (approx. 300 Euros per day), which is covered in part by the sickness funds but in part also by the nursing insurance (Pflegeversicherung). Reimbursement does not cover the whole costs, and the hospices have to raise about 5 per cent of their budget from other funding, mostly charity funding. The positive effect of this reimbursement gap is that hospices have to stay engaged in the local community for charity fundraising.

Patients with complex palliative care needs (complex pain symptoms, respiratory symptoms, neurological or psychiatric symptoms, other complex symptoms) have a right to receive specialized palliative home care (SAPV). This specialized care is free of charge for the patient and the family. The models of care for SAPV differ between the Association of Statutory Health Insurance Physicians (Kassenärztliche Vereinigungen, (KV)), resulting in differences in the service contracts between sickness funds and service providers (and sometimes also KV in trilateral contracts) in the 17 KV regions in Germany.

In most regions, SAPV is provided by multiprofessional teams, consisting of nurses and physicians, sometimes also case manager with palliative care training, and with an option to consult additional expertise, e.g. from psychooncology, physiotherapy, social worker, or spiritual caregiver. Most SAPV contracts describe four levels of specialist palliative home care: consultation (one time), coordination support, partial service, full service. Reimbursements for palliative care delivered by GPs are not possible with the full service level (where the SAPV team is supposed to provide all care), but on all other levels. Reimbursement differs between regions and contracts, and may include flat fees, daily reimbursement rates, or payment per intervention. SAPV is prescribed by the GP for up to 30 days, and this can be repeated as long as needed. The GP has to specify the reason (e.g. complex pain syndrome) and the level of care (e.g. consultation only or full care with around-the-clock availability). When patients are treated as inpatients in hospitals, the treating physician in the hospital can prescribe SAPV for up to seven days after discharge. The GP and the patient have to sign the prescription, which then has to be handed in to the sickness fund within three days. The sickness fund guarantees payment for the first three days, but subsequent payment is subject to approval from the sickness fund.

As this has demonstrated, the system for care is quite complex, but there is a growing support not only from government, but also from other stakeholders, including sickness funds and the German Medical Board for developing care. Palliative care is a mandatory part of the medical curriculum, and ten universities have established a chair for palliative medicine. Palliative care is also part of the nursing curriculum, though with large variations in the extent of teaching between nursing schools.

Woven around this set of care services are volunteers who, as noted previously, provide psychosocial support for patients and their families, but also help raise public awareness of hospices and palliative care through discussing their volunteer engagement with family, friends, and colleagues at work. In this way volunteers working within end-of-life care are facilitating a more open discussion of end of life issues in Germany.

In 2012 the 'Charta zur Versorgung von Schwerstkranken und Sterbenden' (charter for the severly ill and dying), a national joint action led by the German Association for Palliative Medicine, the German Hospice and Palliative Care Society, and the German Medical Association and supported by 1400 organizations and institutions and more than 15,000 individuals (Deutsche Gesellschaft für Palliativmedizin e.V., 2012) was published. This charter acknowledged that volunteering is an expression of citizen engagement and proof of solidarity in society; it acknowledged that volunteering is a core element of hospice work and care for patients and their families, and the charter engages in improving conditions for volunteering.

Developments in palliative care continue as the need is acknowledged from a number of sources. The Leopoldina National Academy of Science prepared and published a research agenda on palliative care, (Nationale Akademie der Wissenschaften Leopoldina and Union der deutschen Akademien der Wissenschaften, 2015) which led to a funding call from the German Ministry of Research for palliative care research proposals in March 2016.

In November 2012 a national media awareness week saw more than 40 television and radio contributions on hospice and palliative care, death, dying, and bereavement, involving patients and both informal and professional caregivers (http://web.ard.de/themenwoche_2012). There have also been a number of documentaries, and some feature films such as 'Halt auf Freier Strecke' (stopped on track), about a patient diagnosed with advanced brain cancer) which raised public awareness.

Within this developing landscape volunteering has been implemented as an integral part of hospice and palliative care. Volunteers consider their contribution to palliative care as essential because they have the feeling that 'they represent society around the dying person and that their work evokes the neighbourly solidarity of the past' (Woitha et al., 2015).

Approaches to management and training

With awareness being raised and a growing number of volunteer services developed as part of the palliative care development in Germany, training programmes for volunteers have been developed and gradually become accepted. (Nationale Akademie der Wissenschaften Leopoldina and Union der deutschen Akademien der Wissenschaften, 2015).

Coordinators of services

As mentioned earlier, coordinators of volunteer services are required to have specific qualifications. Initially, curricula for coordinators were designed to reflect the role of coordinator as the access point and person responsible for volunteer training. The curricula included instructing volunteers in their tasks in hospice palliative care and in communication skills and attitudes. The Celler curriculum was used frequently as a model for local curricula. It was planned for an overall duration of ten to 12 months, including a basic course module of 27 hours, practical training for six to nine months and an advanced course with another 27 hours training.

Volunteers

The Deutscher Hospiz- und Palliativverband (German Hospice and Palliative Care Society) has produced a framework for volunteer work in hospice and palliative care, regulating content, quality and time frame of training (Deutscher Hospiz- und PalliativVerband e.V.). A total of 100 to 120 hours training is recommended. Training should focus first on a reflection on personal motivation, in the second part on qualification and in the final part provide work experience. Volunteer tasks are described in the training as: developing a trusting relationship with the patient, accompanying the patient and the family, giving psychosocial support, dealing with death and dying, facilitating communication, helping with social, ethical, and spiritual issues. The model curriculum includes the themes: communication skills, biography, grief, concept of hospice care, dealing with dying, working in hospice, help the helper, and spirituality. Communication skills are considered to be most important and are the largest part of the curriculum, with exercises in awareness and acceptance, body language, and conversation techniques such as active listening. Biography includes individual experiences with death and dying, influence of philosophy, religion and culture, fear and hope, and emotions. The concept of hospice care explains the history and development of hospice and palliative care, basics of pain management and symptom control, ethical and legal aspects, and tasks of hospice services. Dealing with spirituality necessitates knowledge about religion, symbols, rituals, rites, and ideologies. Volunteers learn about documenting their work, legal regulations of volunteer work, insurance, and public relations. Information and training in self-experience, resilience, and mental hygiene are provided for self-care and prevention of burnout.

Volunteers are also expected to reflect on their role in a multidisciplinary team and their understanding of their volunteer work. Many of the initiatives are faith-bound, though usually they are inclusive of many backgrounds, for the patients they care for the volunteers providing the care. Throughout the training respect for other's attitudes and preferences and the prevention of proselytizing is paramount.

Volunteers' training is a prerequisite for reimbursement of staff costs of the hospice service by the sickness funds—that is to say, that unless volunteers undergo this training, the sickness fund money that goes to funding the coordinator role is not forthcoming. Training is usually provided by the hospice coordinators who manage the hospice services. They also recruit and vet the volunteer candidates, for example excluding people who have lost a loved one only recently, and they also supervise the volunteers in the qualification phase of the training as well as later on after training. The coordinators also make first contact with new patients, assessing their specific needs and preferences. They then match volunteers with patients, plan and coordinate the volunteer involvement with each patient. The coordinators collaborate with other health care providers such as GPs and nursing services.

Why and how volunteering is changing

Hospice and palliative care volunteering is changing in Germany, and this is related to the ongoing development of palliative care on the one hand and to the transition from pioneer phase to integration in mainstream health care on the other hand.

Ongoing development leads to changes in the patient groups that receive palliative care. Palliative care is provided not only to cancer patients, but increasingly patients with chronic heart failure, chronic obstructive pulmonary disease, or neurological diseases obtain access to palliative care as well. There is also a growing number of frail elderly patients, with or without dementia, with hospice and palliative care needs.

These patients have longer disease trajectories with a slower decline in function, and may require hospice care for prolonged periods of time. Where hospice services had tailored their concept of care to the shorter trajectories of cancer patients, they now find that their resources are under pressure as volunteers are involved with these patients for longer than the organization had anticipated. Other approaches may be needed for these patient groups, for example providing high-frequency intensive coverage for short periods of time alternating with expanded periods where the hospice service is on standby. In addition, other skills may be required, for example communication via alphabet board for patients with motor neurone disease. Needs and preferences may differ in these patient groups from those of cancer patients. With hospice and palliative care established in mainstream health care, and growing awareness of hospice and palliative care in the general public, patients and caregivers access the services with high expectations and demands. This and the expected increase in patients requiring palliative care in the next decades due to the demographic change will put big strains on the volunteer services as well as on other hospice and palliative care services.

On the other hand, volunteers themselves are changing. In the beginning of hospice care volunteers were older and often retired middle-class women (Claxton-Oldfield and Banzen, 2010). Now there are also younger people with nine-to-five jobs looking for a meaningful and worthy engagement. These volunteers have less altruistic motivation, but rather seek to collect experience and enhancement of their CV. This also means that these volunteers will work in hospice care for a year or two, in contrast to the much longer times of other volunteers, who often stay engaged in hospice work until they cannot keep it up anymore. For the volunteer services this reduces the return on interest following the investments in training and supervision. It also means that volunteers may initially be attracted to hospice care if there is more public awareness of death and dying, but may also easily shift elsewhere, for example to help with the recent refugee crisis in Germany.

Men are still underrepresented, as volunteering in a caring role traditionally seems to be considered a woman's role. However, crediting social engagement such as hospice volunteering for applications for apprenticeships and study courses provides additional motivation for younger people, and men are becoming open-minded towards this field.

With the development of hospice and palliative care and the concomitant professionalization of volunteers with standardized training and supervision there are also changes in the self-image of volunteering. Curiously enough, this has led to some restrictions in the range of activities. For example, trained volunteers will no longer agree to supervise the patient's application of his medication, which some volunteers had done in the pioneer years. Volunteers certainly will not inject medicines in subcutaneous lines, which has also been done in earlier years. During training they have learned that symptom management and more specifically the application of medicines are medical or nursing tasks, and that they should not get involved, as there may be liability issues. Similarly, some volunteers will not do household activities such as cleaning or shopping for the patient, as they have been trained to focus on the psychosocial support of patient and caregivers. With the ongoing development volunteers become more professional, but this results in a loss of flexibility, as volunteer tasks get narrowed down and streamlined.

In some cases, new roles and tasks are emerging for volunteers. For example, palliative care training is mandatory for medical students, even though there is no specific curriculum for this topic. In our university we have 14 hours of small group education in addition to 14 hours of lectures. Small group work includes sessions with actor patients, among others. A number of interested volunteers have been trained to act as simulated patients. They can translate their experiences with similar situations in their volunteer work in realistic encounters with the medical students. We are currently planning to expand this training with actor patients to the training courses for physicians and nurses.

In Germany, with the integration of palliative care into mainstream health care, an increasing amount of competition and economic pressure has been introduced. Palliative care and hospice services have to compete with other health care services for resources, and different palliative care and hospice services in a region start competing for patients and charity funding. Even if the new hospice and palliative care law requires formal collaboration of nursing homes and hospitals with volunteer services, effective implementation of these collaborations requires the mutual trust of all collaborators.

Similarly, the integration of basic and specialist palliative care in local and regional palliative care networks requires trust and high transparency. The complexity of the networks is increasing, with GPs, oncologists, but also nursing home staff becoming interested and starting to provide hospice and palliative care. New players in the field, such as GPs setting up palliative care networks or newly established specialist palliative home care teams, have an impact on volunteer services. They often lack information about the tasks and resources of the volunteer services and thus will not include their services in the patient's care plan. Volunteer coordinators, who sometimes have been the local pioneers and have been a focus point for the provision of hospice and palliative care, may feel pushed aside by new specialist services that try to take over the coordination of hospice and palliative care in the region. Volunteers suddenly find themselves in a for-profit segment of health care and face competition from other services. Families sometimes feel overburdened with too many persons from different services coming to their aid, and they may try to restrict the number of care providers. These changes may lead to an alienation of services instead of the construction of effective and integrated networks. All these changes may require a revision of the role of volunteers in palliative and hospice care.

Factors that contribute to success

When discussing the development of volunteering in Germany terminology has to be considered (Radbruch et al., 2015). The German term for volunteering is 'Ehrenamt' (honorary office). Some communities have 'Ehrenamt-Börsen' (honorary office market) to link interested persons with services. Alternatively 'Bürgerschaftliches Engagement (civic engagement) is used in the political context. Using this terminology associates both honour and official status to volunteering, making it seem nobler than with the volunteer term alone.

On the other hand, volunteering in Germany is not as self-evident as it is in other countries. The well-developed social security and insurance system has led to an underlying attitude that people are entitled to support from the health care system for the problems they encounter. The claim for full support devaluates volunteer contributions.

The main motivation for people seeking engagement in hospice care is altruism. In a German volunteer survey in 2015 (Katherina Pabst, personal communication) the top five motivations were: 1. belief that everyone should give something back to the community, 2. the wish to make others comfortable in life, as well as until death, 3. help others cope with death and dying, 4. help those who are facing death, and 5. responsibility to help others. The least-rated motivations were: 1. to improve the image portrayed to family, friends, and society, 2. hobby, 3. people tend to look favourably on volunteers, 4. requirement to fulfil ones involvement in another activity, and 5. generally people are obligated to provide service to the towns they live in.

Recent developments in volunteering in Germany include a new focus on bereavement support. This is a unique selling point of volunteer services. Grief is not in the focus of health care professionals until it becomes complex. Volunteer services offer low-level interventions, for example bereavement cafés, bereavement groups, or individual consultations, and many of the volunteers have been trained in bereavement support. With these, activities volunteer services have taken over a field that is an integral part of hospice and palliative care, but is not covered by the health care system. This provides volunteer services with an opportunity to strengthen their position in the field.

Conclusion

Volunteering in hospice and palliative care does provide a benefit both for the volunteers and the hospice and palliative care services. Volunteers get a reward and see a value in their work. They have no fixed agenda; they can comply with the individual wishes of the patient. Their core competencies are flexibility, communication on eye level, and connecting patients with normal daily life. Services benefit from the time the volunteers dedicate. Volunteers bear testimony to the solidarity of the community and they convey humanity and dignity to the severely ill and dying. With due consideration of these essential arguments volunteers are indispensable for hospice and palliative care services.

References

Aulbert, E., Albrecht, H., Nauck, F., and Radbruch, L. (2012) *Lehrbuch der Palliativmedizin: mit* 2012) 5. Aufl. *204 Tabellen*, Stuttgart: Schattauer.

Bundesgesetzblatt. (2015) *Bundesgesetzblatt Teil I, Nr. 48 vom 07.12.2015, Gesetz zur Verbesserung der Hospiz- und Palliativversorgung in Deutschland (Hospiz- und Palliativgesetz-HPG)* [Online]. Available from: http://www.bgbl.de/xaver/bgbl/start. xav?startbk=Bundesanzeiger_BGBl&jumpTo=bgbl115s2114.pdf [Accessed 23.05.2016.]

Claxton-Oldfield, S. and Banzen, Y. (2010) Personality characteristics of hospice palliative care volunteers: the 'big five' and empathy. *Am J Hosp Palliat Care* 27(6): 407–12.

Deutsche Gesellschaft für Palliativmedizin E.V. (2012) Charta zur Betreuung schwerstkranker und sterbender Menschen in Deutschland (2012) 5. Aufl.

Deutscher Bundestag 15. Wahlperiode (2005). *Zwischenbericht der Enquete-Kommission Ethik und Recht der modernen Medizin, Verbesserung der Versorgung Schwerstkranker und Sterbender in Deutschland durch Palliativmedizin und Hospizarbeit* [Online]. Available from: http://dipbt.bundestag.de/doc/btd/15/058/1505858.pdf [Accessed 22.08.2012.]

Deutscher Hospiz-und PalliativVerband E.V (2010). *Rahmenvereinbarung nach § 39a Abs. 2 Satz 7 SGB V zu den Voraussetzungen der Förderung sowie zu Inhalt, Qualität und*

Umfang der ambulanten Hospizarbeit vom 03.09.2002, i. d. F. vom 14.04.2010 [Online]. Available from: http://www.dhpv.de/tl_files/public/Service/Gesetze%20und%20 Verordnungen/amb_rahmen_p39a-sgb5.pdf.

Economist Intelligence Unit. (2015) *The quality of death. Ranking end-of-life care across the world* [Online]. Available from: http://www.economistinsights.com/healthcare/analysis/ quality-death-index-2015 [Accessed 1.3.2016.]

Melching, H. (2015) *Palliativversorgung Modul 2: Strukturen und regionale Unterschiede in der Hospiz- und Palliativversorgung,* Gütersloh: Bertelsmann Stiftung.

Nationale Akademie der Wissenschaften Leopoldina & Union Der Deutschen Akademien Der Wissenschaften. (2015) Palliativversorgung in Deutschland—Perspektiven für Praxis und Forschung. Available from: http://www.leopoldina.org/uploads/tx_ leopublication/2015_Palliativversorgung_LF_DE.pdf [Accessed 30.5.2015.]

Radbruch, L., Hesse, M., Pelttari, L., and Scott, R. (2015) *The Full Range of Volunteering: Views on Palliative Care Volunteering from seven countries.* Bonn: Pallia Med.

Woitha, K., Hasselaar, J., Van Beek, K., Radbruch, L., Jaspers, B., Engels, Y., and Vissers, K. (2015) Volunteers in palliative care—A comparison of seven European countries: A descriptive study. *Pain Pract* **15**(6): 572–9.

Worldwide Palliative Care Alliance. 2014. Global Atlas of Palliative Care at the end of life. Available from: http://www.who.int/nmh/Global_Atlas_of_Palliative_Care.pdf

Chapter 7

Volunteering in hospice and palliative care in Poland and Eastern Europe

Piotr Krakowiak and Leszek Pawłowski

The solidarity of volunteers: the beginning of the hospice movement in Poland

Poland is one of the largest countries in Central-Eastern Europe and, according to the recent data from EAPC Atlas of Palliative Care in Europe, for many years it has held a leading role in the whole region (Clark and Centeno, 2006; Centeno et al., 2013). In Poland, as in most of Europe, hospices for the seriously ill and dying had existed for centuries, usually run by Christian orders and fraternities (Przygoda, 2004). The impetus for what we see as palliative care today came in the 1970s in Cracow when the Catholic Church was looking for new ways to serve. There, one of the synod groups of the archdiocese appointed by Cardinal Karol Wojtyła (future Pope John Paul II), set up a group of volunteers willing to help the dying and their families. The impetus and inspiration came to this gathering of volunteers through Dame Cicely Saunders whose visit is reflected in official writings on the beginnings of hospice care: 'The beginnings of the development of hospice and palliative care in Poland date back to 1978, when the first lectures on these issues were given in Poland by Cicely Saunders, the founder of the first modern hospice' (Ministry of Health and Social Welfare, 1998: 1). In 1981 the first hospice association in Eastern Europe was set up which was also the first Polish independent charity organization based on the work of volunteers. They chose Dame Cicely's St. Christopher's Hospice in London as model. Development during the years of political difficulties and democratic transformations however, meant the Cracow hospice was only opened as the inpatient hospice in 1996 (Janowicz et al., 2015). A second centre of care for the dying was the Home Care Hospice established in Gdańsk in 1983. Interestingly, the impetus came through a group active in the Gdańsk 'Solidarność' Union Healthcare Section, supported by the chaplain of the Medical University of

Gdańsk Father Eugeniusz Dutkiewicz, and a professor, Joanna Muszkowska-Penson MD, PhD (Krakowiak and Stolarczyk, 2007). Their actions came in spite of the bans imposed by the authorities and martial law. The communist regime was losing support, and the initiatives to improve the end of life care came from the Church and Solidarity—both critical of state power. In effect, something as 'fundamental' as end of life care sprung at least in part from 'the opposition' to state power. Doctors, medical students, and representatives of other professions decided to act against the existing system of care and were reaching out as volunteers to people dying at home without adequate medical care (Janowicz et al., 2015: 35). Meetings and training courses provided information and education about hospice home care, which, given the situation of the country at that time, was the optimum model of care for people towards the end of their life (Krakowiak and Janowicz, 2013). The Hospice in Gdańsk had its roots in the ideals of Solidarity, born in this city and having direct support of its leader, Lech Wałęsa and others from Solidarity Movement.

The beginning of transformation and integration in hospice and palliative care in Poland

The significance of a volunteer-led hospice service in local communities was not lost on the Ministry of Health and Social Welfare which noted that: 'The hospice teams forming in many towns were organized as informal groups or as church or secular associations with their own statutes. The primary form of care is hospice home care provided by physicians, nurses, a chaplain and a psychologist totally free of charge, with their own means of transport lent for home visits' (Ministry of Health and Social Welfare, 1998: p. 1–2). Here then was a community-led activity which as well as providing services was raising social awareness and educating wider society about the needs of the terminally ill. The problems of dying and death, practically absent from the mass media, were not included in the education of health care and social welfare employees at that time. Those groups of volunteers in local communities made use of the already developed concept of hospice care, even under communism in 1988, patients and families in Poland were taken care of in home centres run by volunteers (Janowicz et al., 2015: 38).

In parallel with the social and *spiritual* hospice movement based on volunteers in Poland, the *science* of palliative care had started to develop with a group of medical professionals in Poznań in 1987, who started work modelling themselves on the Milan palliative medicine centre. Around the same time, just before the democratic changes in 1989, a National Hospice Chaplain had been appointed by the Catholic Bishops' Conference. Soon the hospice and palliative care teams operating at the time in Poland, formed a common body together with the first physicians trained internationally in palliative care. Eventually, in 1993, integration of hospice and palliative care in Poland developed further with the appointment of the National Council for Palliative and Hospice Care at the Ministry of Health and Social Welfare, which invited the participation of representatives of communities associated with the voluntary hospice movement and palliative medicine specialists. By 1998, 'The Program of Development of Palliative and Hospice Care in Poland' was approved and the inclusion of hospice and palliative care in the law on health care and social care facilities contributed to the total incorporation of the social movement in health care and welfare structures, which was at that time unique in the whole of Eastern Europe (Janowicz et al., 2015: 38). Today among East-Central Europe, Poland, and Romania represent the highest level of palliative care development, which, in consequence promotes volunteering (Lynch et al., 2013).

Others followed from the Polish example; in the 1990s, representatives from the region took part in a series of meetings and training organized by Professor Jacek Łuczak, from the Palliative Care Department in Poznań. The significance of the Poznań centre and its leading position in Eastern and Central Europe was confirmed when it was awarded the status of the registered seat of the Eastern and Central European Palliative Care Task Force (ECEPT) in 1999. Even as Poland led the way across the region expertise was continuing to develop in the country with palliative medicine for doctors and palliative care for nurses becoming new areas of professional specialization (Janowicz et al., 2015: 40).

In concluding this brief history it is useful to emphasize that even under communism Polish volunteers created over 80 hospice home care teams. By 1998 Poland was leading Central and Eastern Europe in including hospice and palliative care in health care systems. According to recent data from the EAPC Atlas of Palliative Care in Europe (Centeno et al., 2013: 235) there are now more than 400 different centres of hospice and palliative care in Poland, most of them involving volunteers.

Different statutes of volunteering in hospice and palliative care in changing Eastern Europe

Although Poland may have been a beacon for palliative care it is by no means true that there is as a result one model in the region. Instead, a considerable variety of volunteering in hospice and palliative care in Central and Eastern European countries is evident largely as a result of diverse political, economic, and legal situations, and we can identify two main determinants: 1) the state of palliative care, being closely related to volunteering (i.e. the higher number of hospices and the better level of palliative care services, the more volunteers involved), 2) the accession of some countries to the European Union (EU). It is important to note that the history of the region means that there is generally a lower rate of volunteering in post-communist countries than in North and Western Europe (Plagnol and Huppert, 2010).

Post 1989, the advent of democracy and the free market has meant most East European countries have undergone significant changes in legal and political systems. Gone are the political restrictions on assembling, the foundation of non-governmental organizations, and the undertaking of grassroots initiatives. These changes have all contributed positively to volunteering development (Krakowiak, 2015: 21). Nevertheless, along with the previously mentioned positive changes, the health and social care systems have had to deal with new challenges such as poverty and unemployment, (Saltman and Figueras, 1996). It is a familiar story of non-governmental organizations and churches with the help of volunteers stepping in to deal with many of the issues the state and market cannot (Łuczak, 1993).

Before 1989 volunteering was not as prevalent in the region as it was in Western Europe (Voicu and Voicu, 2009). In the 1990s, hospice and palliative care centres helped lead the way for volunteering which grew rapidly with inter-disciplinary teams which included professionals performing their activities as volunteers (Fürst, 2002; Radbruch, et al., 2014). The incorporation of palliative care into health care systems brought financing which led to the employment of paid staff changing the nature of the voluntary sector so that the number of professionals working as volunteers has radically decreased (Krakowiak, 2015: 21). In turn this means volunteers tend to be those without any specific qualifications, while the majority of physicians, nurses, psychologists, and physiotherapists became paid employees (Pawłowski et al., 2016). Volunteering today is thus less involved in medical care and more about supporting roles such as: accompanying patients, feeding, dressing and bathing them, cleaning rooms and facilities, organizing leisure time, charity work and fundraising, and involvement in providing information and education relating to hospice activity (Pawłowski et al., 2016).

As the nature of volunteering changed so new initiatives were launched to increase awareness of volunteering and palliative care. In 2003 the Hospice Foundation in Gdańsk started to support volunteering and its promotion, aimed at disseminating good practices of cooperation among professionals and volunteers (Krakowiak, 2015: Łuczak and Hunter, 2000). In 2007–10 the Hospice Foundation introduced a project promoting hospice volunteering called 'I like helping' across 100 hospices in Poland. The project was aimed at volunteer coordinators, (some paid, some unpaid), who took part in training and specialist meetings as well as having the opportunity to take advice from experts in volunteering (Hospice Foundation, 2013). In 2006 the Hospice Foundation set out a pioneering programme 'WHAT' (translated as Hospice Voluntary Work as a Tool of Acceptance and Tolerance for People Leaving Penal Institutions) involving prisoners as hospice volunteers (Krakowiak et al., 2013). Ten Polish hospices permanently engaged prisoners as volunteers, which turned out to be beneficial for both parties (Krakowiak and Paczkowska, 2014). One study indicated that participation improves prisoners' psychosocial functioning and their work as hospice volunteers increases the quality of care (Krakowiak et al., 2013). On the basis of the Hospice Foundation experience, The Order of Nurses Midwives and Medical Assistants in Romania (OAMGMAMR) has produced a programme to acquire and adapt international models of good practice in volunteering in hospice and palliative care. The implementation of this project may have a relevant impact on introducing universal standards to voluntary work in palliative care settings (OAMGMAMR, 2015).

Another factor that affected the development of volunteering is the accession of the Czech Republic, Estonia, Hungary, Latvia, Lithuania, Poland, Slovakia, (2004) as well as Bulgaria and Romania (2007) to the European Union (EU). The EU policy is broadly favourable to the development of volunteering and many projects and programmes are a source of additional funds for such enterprises. This, in turn, may cover the costs of a wide variety of activities related to the promotion of volunteering and volunteers' training. On the other hand, countries which are not members of the EU, such as Belarus, Russia, and Ukraine do not have this kind of support, and consequently the development of volunteering in palliative care there is growing much more slowly (Lynch et al., 2009).

Legislative and political influences on volunteering

Policy and law across the region concerning volunteering is diverse. In the Czech Republic, Hungary, Lithuania, Latvia, Moldova, Poland, Romania, and Slovakia the principles of volunteering are precisely regulated by the law (Czech Republic, 2002; Hungary, 2005; Lithuania, 2011; Latvia, 2015; Moldova, 2010; Poland, 2003; Romania, 2014; Slovakia, 2014). On the other hand, there is no legislation on volunteering in Belarus, Bulgaria, Estonia, and Ukraine. In some countries, such as Russia, the law is limited to selected issues, such as the definition of the volunteer and the reimbursement of expenses for volunteering (Russia, 1995). Elsewhere, interested parties campaign to establish legal regulations, for example Bulgaria has developed a draft act in that respect (Ministry of Youth and Sports, 2011).

Legal regulations tend to define the fundamental principles of volunteering, but not its particular forms (e.g. volunteering in hospitals, fundraising, volunteering on phone helplines, etc.). Obviously, these regulations also apply to volunteering in hospice and palliative care, although they are not the only ones regulating this type of service. Additional regulations are also present in a given country, and include patients' rights, occupational health and safety, as well as protection from infections and infectious diseases.

Broadly speaking, the legal definitions across countries define a volunteer as a person who voluntarily provides services and does not receive any remuneration for it. In general, the volunteers' activities are performed within non-profit organizations, that are named, depending on the country, as beneficiary, delegating organization, host organization, or volunteer organization (Poland, 2003; Czech Republic, 2002; Hungary, 2005; Lithuania, 2011). In hospice and palliative care, volunteers usually give their services both to the centre and to the patients and their families. Also volunteers may work as volunteer coordinators, which has been especially included in Romanian law (Romania, 2014).

There are some differences in Central and Eastern European countries regarding minimum age for volunteers; in Hungary the age is ten years, Lithuania and Moldova 14, the Czech Republic and Slovakia 15, and in Latvia the volunteer must be at least 16 years old. Other countries do not indicate any age restrictions. Nevertheless, there may be other laws or regulations depending on services which volunteers carry out, for example where there may be issues around the protection of patients. An interesting comment regarding young volunteers is present in Hungarian law, which it states: 'A person under 18 years of age, or an adult with restricted legal capacity may pursue public interest volunteer activities that correspond to his/her age, physical, mental and moral development and abilities, and do not constitute a risk to his/her health, development and performance of school attendance obligations' (Hungary, 2005: p. 4).

The involvement of volunteers is associated with the need to keep relevant documentation such as agreements, declarations, or databases. In most cases, centres which benefit from volunteering determine the record-keeping system of this data. However, in Latvia, Moldova, Slovakia, and Hungary the obligation to register volunteers and the types of data to be collected is regulated by law.

According to legislation, the cooperation between the volunteer and the palliative care centre should be based on an agreement which is concluded verbally or in writing. The latter form is required usually in the case of long-term contracts (Hungary—over ten days, Poland—more than 30 days, the Czech Republic—more than three months), or for an indefinite period (e.g. Hungary). In Lithuania, Latvia, and Poland, the volunteer may request the confirmation of the oral agreement in writing. Moreover, Lithuanian and Latvian law always requires the written form of the agreement in cases where expenses are reimbursed, and in Latvia even if the volunteer is under 18. In Moldova the written agreement with the volunteer is required when he or she works at least 20 hours a month.

In accordance with the law, the voluntary service agreement should include the following elements: identification of the parties, their rights and duties, volunteer services, duration of the agreement, and the place of provision of the voluntary services. Additionally, in Moldova, Poland, Romania, Slovakia, and Hungary, the agreement should include information how to terminate it, which is crucial in resignation from volunteering. In the Czech Republic, Moldova, and Romania the agreement should also include the volunteers' qualifications, their skills, and information about their health, which may be essential in recruiting patient-facing volunteers. In Moldova, the agreement specifies the scope of volunteers' responsibilities as well as describing the property entrusted to the volunteer.

Volunteers' rights and duties are not only moral obligations, but are also enshrined in legislation. The most common rights that are enumerated in the law of individual countries include the right to:

1. Information about the performed services
2. Information about rights and duties
3. Information about the risks to health and safety and on protection
4. Work in a healthy and safety environment
5. Refuse to perform some activities ordered by a superior
6. The provision of appropriate orientation and training
7. Rest
8. Receive a certificate confirming voluntary activities ·
9. Resign from volunteering
10. Reimbursement of agreed expenses

Here are the responsibilities of the volunteers on the basis of selected legislation (from Hungary, Lithuania, Latvia, Moldova, and Romania). Volunteers are obliged to:

1. Perform assigned tasks and orders of superiors
2. Perform their services in accordance with legal regulations, ethical principles, and internal rules set by the organization as well as the agreement
3. Perform their services personally
4. Maintain confidentiality about patients, their families, and the organization

5. Care for the property of the organization and the property entrusted to the volunteer

The main characteristic feature of voluntary work is that there is no financial gain. Obviously, the costs associated with provision of services must not be considered as remuneration. In most countries, national law provides the possibility of covering such costs. In the Czech Republic, Latvia, Lithuania, Moldova, and Slovakia the voluntary agreement may include the rules of reimbursement. In Romania, the beneficiary organization has an obligation to cover such costs, and in Poland, travel expenses and daily subsistence allowance must be paid.

The insurance of volunteers is a much more complicated and diverse issue in light of the policies of various countries. In general, the hospice may provide the accident insurance and liability insurance for the volunteer (in Hungary it is an obligation). In Poland, in the case of an accident, each volunteer can benefit from insurance, which is ensured by the country or by the centre (depending on the period for which the agreement was signed). In Romania, the insurance is arranged on the request of the volunteer. In Moldova, Poland, and Slovakia the centre can provide volunteer health insurance, and in the Czech Republic and Slovakia, pension insurance.

Czech, Lithuanian, Moldovan, Romanian, and Slovak law requires the beneficiary organization to ensure training for the volunteer candidates is provided to prepare them for their tasks; in the other countries it is not law so much as good practice. Romanian law goes further to include a detailed proposed course content, consisting of: information about the structure and activities carried out by the beneficiary organization, the volunteers' rights and duties, and the internal rules referring to the involvement of volunteers. According to the legal regulations of most countries, volunteers perform activities corresponding to their qualifications and skills. This requirement also takes account of volunteers' health, especially in the case of those working directly with patients. Another requirement, which should be taken into account during recruiting potential volunteers is the presence of criminal history, which in the Czech Republic and Latvia has been included in their law. According to the legislation in these countries such people cannot be volunteers.

In countries in which volunteering has not been regulated by law, its conditions are set individually by the organization and the volunteer. Thus, the agreement between the parties is signed on general principles of civil law. In countries which have regulations concerning the protection of patients' rights, the patient-facing volunteers must fulfill a number of criteria. For example, in Poland a volunteers in hospice and palliative care must follow the patients' rights to: respect for intimacy and dignity, die in peace and dignity, maintain confidentiality of information related to the patient, respect the will of the patient, as well as their preferences for contact with other people. The volunteer carries liability for violation of these rights (Poland, 2008). In effect, in most Central and Eastern European countries the volunteer is responsible for any harm caused to the patient. In contrast, in Moldova and Hungary (with few exceptions) the institution is responsible. Liability insurance for the volunteer, which the hospice may ensure, may protect the volunteer from financial responsibility.

Factors contributing to success of hospice and palliative care volunteering in Eastern Europe

Volunteering in hospice and palliative care in Central and Eastern European countries has developed within a similar historical context, but under diverse political, social, and economic conditions. Its development has been determined both by external factors (benefitting from the experiences of others, membership of the EU) and also internal determinants. The latter includes society's perception of volunteering; the state of hospice and palliative care; its financing by national health insurance; the engagement of state and local authorities; assistance of religious institutions, and legal regulations concerning volunteering as the presence of organizations which support the development of volunteering in palliative care, and the training of its members and coordinators. Important also is the cooperation of hospices with all kinds of authorities, foundations, churches, and means of mass communication that may bring about the promotion of volunteering, funds for its activities, and volunteer recruitment. Not least, we must also view the condition of volunteering in particular countries as a factor of their economic growth and society's standard of living (Prouteau and Sardinha, 2011). Therefore, volunteering in palliative care is at a higher level in countries which are members of the EU and benefit from its financial support, than that of non-EU members (Voicu and Voicu, 2009).

In 2013, in the Czech Republic there were 15 residential hospices and four mobile hospices and each of them benefitted from the help of ten to 60 volunteers trained in hospice and palliative care (Spinkova, 2013). In Lithuania, thanks to the support of St. Luke's Hospice (London) and the British Embassy in Vilnius, special training programmes for volunteers were introduced. According to the report from 2012, this education produced a progression within the state of the development of palliative care centres and volunteering (Coward, 2012). Similarly, in 2012 Romania implemented a programme including models of good practice based on other countries' experiences, called 'Volunteering in palliative care in Romania', which aims to prepare 40 volunteer coordinators to organize volunteering in palliative care settings (OAMGMAMR, 2015). The major Russian success story is the foundation and activity of Hospice Charity Fund Vera, which provides financial support for 30 hospices. The foundation also carries out activities devoted to palliative care, such as an educational programme which is focused on attracting more volunteers to hospices all over Russia. As a result of this programme, a team of over 400 volunteers was developed and maintained in 2015 (VERA Hospice Charity Fund, 2015).

In Ukraine the foundation of the Ukrainian Palliative and Hospice Care League was formed in 2011. Its priority is the development of the volunteer movement and implementing training programmes on palliative care for volunteers (Ukrainian Palliative and Hospice Care League, 2013). In countries such as Lithuania, Latvia, Moldova, Romania, and Slovakia an important factor in improving conditions for the development of volunteering has been the recent introduction of a law for volunteering. Indeed, in countries which do not have such legislation, as e.g. Belarus, the lack of adequate legislation may cause some doubt and uncertainty about the involvement of volunteers in hospices (Spasiuk, 2008).

New challenges for end of life care volunteering in Eastern Europe

Fast-ageing societies of Poland and Eastern Europe require social education and the promotion of volunteers in local communities. Demographic changes and the growing number of chronically ill and old people living alone in their homes call for specific actions to be taken. In view of the necessity to support people in need of assistance at home and their family members caring for them, some teams in Poland have started to cooperate with the Roman-Catholic charitable organization Caritas, in order to establish voluntary services for chronically ill and elderly people in local communities nearing the end of life. Thus, the knowledge and experience of hospice and palliative care can be transferred to the difficult realities of home care in Poland and in other countries of Eastern Europe. Successful examples of such a transfer of good practices have been noted in Poland. These have been implemented by means of publications, lectures, and workshops with guidebooks for families and volunteers as home care assistants. Experts from hospice and palliative care have prepared a set of books for volunteers and families: 'The Chronically Ill at Home' (2010 and 2011), 'Voluntary Service in End-of-Life Care' (2012) and 'The Art of Communication with the Terminally Ill' (2013 and 2014) (Krakowiak, 2015).

Hospice and palliative care centres in Poland could become educational and training centres for professionals and volunteers providing care for people in their own homes.

Recruitment, training, and coordination of volunteers could also be developed in local communities on the basis of over 30 years' experience of the hospice palliative care services, teamwork, and volunteering coordination.

The introduction of good practices in teamwork with volunteers into long-term care, social welfare and, above all, home care, through academic and educational actions in local communities presents another opportunity and challenge. East European societies, which are the fastest ageing societies in the European Union, with many young people still migrating to the West, need the further education of professionals and volunteers, international cooperation, research, and the exchange of good practices in end of life care. Without losing the hospice spirit which helped to start end of life care in Poland and other parts of Eastern Europe years ago (Krakowiak et al., 2016: 603), the courage to share it with families and other professionals of health and social care is needed. There are challenges here, but solidarity and experiences of teamwork and the cooperation of professionals and volunteers give us hope in reaching more of those who need help in the last stage of their life.

References

Centeno, C., Lynch, T., Donea, O., Rocafort, J., and Clark, D. (2013) *EAPC Atlas of Palliative Care in Europe*. Full (ed.) pp. 235–41. Available from: http://dadun.unav.edu/handle/10171/29291?locale=en [Accessed 25.11.2016.]

Clark, D, and Centeno, C. (2006) Palliative care in Europe: an emerging approach to comparative analysis. *Clinical Medicine (London)* 6(2): 197–201.

Coward, M. (2012) There is no official word for 'hospice' in Lithuanian. Available from: http://thetiltastrust.org/wp-content/uploads/2012/11/Mike-Cowards-Report-August-2012-MJP.pdf [Accessed 30.07.2016.]

Czech Republic (2002) Act of 24 April 2002 on Volunteer Services, no. 198.

Fürst, C. (2002) The European Association for Palliative Care initiative in Eastern Europe. *Journal of Pain and Symptom Management* 24(2): 134–5.

Hospice Foundation (2013) *Brief history*. Available from: http://www.fundacjahospicyjna.pl/en/about-us/brief-history [Accessed 30.07.2016.]

Hungary (2005) Act on Public Interest Volunteer Activities 2005, no. LXXXVIII.

Krakowiak, P. (2015) Emergence of the contemporary hospice movement in Poland. In *Solidarity*, pp. 32–9. (ed.) Janowicz, A., Krakowiak, P., and Stolarczyk, A., Poland: Fundacja Hospicyjna.

Krakowiak, P. (2015) Special role and forms of voluntary service in hospice-palliative care in Poland. In *Solidarity* pp. 46–62. (ed.) Janowicz, A., Krakowiak, P., and Stolarczyk, A., Poland: Fundacja Hospicyjna.

Krakowiak, P. and Janowicz, A. (2013) *The History of the Pallottine Hospice in Gdańsk—Thirty years in the service of dying 1983-2013.* pp. 31–5. Poland: Fundacja Hospicyjna.

Krakowiak, P. and Paczkowska, A. (2014) Włączanie skazanych do wolontariatu opieki paliatywno-hospicyjnej na świecie i w Polsce. Dobre praktyki współpracy systemu penitencjarnego ze środowiskiem opieki paliatywno-hospicyjnej w Polsce, *Probacja* (2): 47–64.

Krakowiak, P., and Stolarczyk, A. ed. (2007) *Father Eugeniusz Dutkiewicz SAC. Father of Hospice Movement in Poland*, pp. 78–9. Poland: Fundacja Hospicyjna.

Krakowiak, P., Paczkowska, A., and Witkowski, R. (2013) Prisoners as hospice volunteers in Poland. *Medycyna Paliatywna w Praktyce* **7**(2): 55–64.

Krakowiak P. (2015) Hospice—Palliative care volunteering in Poland as a resource for others in Central—Eastern Europe. Available from: http://www.hospiz.at/pdf_dl/Volunteering_PL_PKrakowiak.pdf [Accessed 30.07.2016.]

Krakowiak, P. (2015) Keeping the Hospice Spirit Alive. In *In Solidarity* p. 104, (ed.) Janowicz, A., Krakowiak, P., and Stolarczyk, A., Poland: Fundacja Hospicyjna.

Krakowiak, P. (2015) Then and now. In *In Solidarity* pp. 21–66, (ed.) Janowicz, A., Krakowiak, P., and Stolarczyk, A., Poland: Fundacja Hospicyjna.

Krakowiak, P., Skrzypinska, K., Damps-Konstanska, I., and Jassem, E. (2016) Walls and Barriers. Polish achievements and the challenges of transformation: Building a hospice movement in Poland. *Journal of Pain and Symptom Management* **52**(4): 600–604.

Latvia (2015) Act of 18 June 2015 on Volunteering, no. 127.1.

Leppert, W. (2015) A Doctor's Reflections after 20 Years of Work at an Academic Palliative Medicine Centre. In *In Solidarity*. pp. 117–22, (ed.) Janowicz, A., Krakowiak, P., and Stolarczyk, A., Poland: Fundacja Hospicyjna.

Lithuania (2011) Republic of Lithuania Law on Volunteering 2011, no. XI-1500.

Luczak, J. and Hunter, G. (2000) Hospice care in eastern Europe. *Lancet* Suppl. **356**: 23.

Luczak, J. (1993) Palliative/hospice care in Poland. *Palliative Medicine* **7**(1): 67–75.

Lynch, T., Clark, D., Centeno, C., Rocafort, J., Flores, L., Greenwooda, A., Praill, D., Brasch, S., Giordano, A., De Lima, L., and Wright, M. (2009) Barriers to the development of palliative care in the countries of Central and Eastern Europe and the Commonwealth of Independent States, *Journal of Pain and Symptom Management* **37**(3): 305–15. doi: 10.1016/j.jpainsymman.2008.03.011.

Lynch, T., Connor, S., and Clark, D. (2013) Mapping levels of palliative care development: a global update. *Journal of Pain and Symptom Management* **45**(6): 1094–106.

Ministry of Health and Social Welfare (1998) *Program of Development of Palliative and Hospice Care in Poland*, p. 1. Poland.

Ministry of Youth and Sports (2011) Draft Law on Volunteering. Available from: http://mc.government.bg/files/1174-_Dobrovolchestvo.doc [Accessed 30.07.2016.]

Moldova (2010) Act of 18 June 2010 on Volunteering, no. 121/2010.

Pawłowski, L., Lichodziejewska-Niemierko, M., Pawłowska, I., Leppert, W., and Mróz, P. (2016) Nationwide survey on volunteers' training in hospice and palliative care in Poland. *BMJ Supportive and Palliative Care*, Published Online First: 29 July 2016. doi: 10.1136/bmjspcare-2015-000984.

Plagnol, A. and Huppert, F.(2010) Happy to Help? Exploring the Factors Associated with Variations in Rates of Volunteering Across Europe. *Social Indicators Research* **97**(2): 157–76, doi: 10.1007/s11205-009-9494-x.

Poland (2003) Act of 24 April 2003 on Public Benefit and Volunteer Work.

Poland (2008) Act of 6 November 2008 on Patients' Rights and Patients' Rights Ombudsman.

Prouteau, L. and **Sardinha, B.** (2011) European volunteering: comparisons, individual and country determinants. Available from: https://comum.rcaap.pt/bitstream/10400.26/ 5311/1/Paper-Prouteau-Sardinha_ERNOP%5B2%5D.pdf [Accessed 30.07.2016.]

Przygoda, W. (2004) *Charitable Service of the Church in Poland. A theological and pastoral study*, pp. 167–8. Poland: Wydawnictwo Katolickiego Uniwersytetu Lubelskiego.

Radbruch, L., Hesse, M., Pelttari, L., and Scott R. ed. (2014) *The full range of Volunteering, Views on Palliative Care Volunteering from seven countries as gathered in March 2014 in Bonn*. Germany: Pallia Med Verlag.

Romania (2014) Act regarding the Regulation of the Volunteering Activity 2014, no. 78/ 2014.

Russia (1995) Federal law on charitable activities and organizations, 1995, no. 135-fz.

Saltman, R. and **Figueras, G.** (1996) *European Health Care Reform: Analysis of Current Strategies*. WHO Regional Office for Europe, WHO, 23 April 1996. Available from: http://www.euro.who.int/__data/assets/pdf_file/0005/111011/sumhecareform. pdf. [Accessed 30.07.2016.]

Slovakia (2014) Act on volunteering and on amendment of certain laws 2014, no. 406/2011.

Spasiuk, E. (2008) *Belarus should have the law on volunteering*. Available from: http://naviny. by/rubrics/society/2008/12/05/ic_articles_116_160227. [Accessed 30.07.2016.]

Spinkova, M. (2013) *Ordinary or Peculiar Folk? On the Role of Volunteers in Palliative Care in Czech Republic*. Available from: http://www.eapcnet.eu/LinkClick.aspx?fileticket=cW QnXUT0Ado%3Dandtabid=1913. [Accessed 30.07.2016.]

The Order of Nurses Midwives and Medical Assistants in Romania (2015) *Volunteering in palliative care in Romania*. Available from: http://oamrsm.ro/?p=2335. [Accessed 30.07.2016.]

Ukrainian Palliative and Hospice Care League (2013) *Our objectives*. Available from: http:// en.ligalife.com.ua/108/. [Accessed 30.07.2016.]

VERA Hospice Charity Fund (2015) *Someone who can't be cured can still be helped.* Available from: http://www.hospicefund.ru/wp-content/uploads/2015/02/In_English. pdf. [Accessed 30.07.2016.]

Voicu, B. and **Voicu, M.** (2009) Volunteers and volunteering in Central and Eastern Europe. *Sociológia* **41**(6): 539–63.

Chapter 8

Volunteering in hospice palliative care in Canada

Stephen Claxton-Oldfield

Brief history of hospice palliative care volunteering in Canada

The development of formalized hospice palliative care began with the opening of hospital-based palliative care units at the St. Boniface General Hospital in Winnipeg, Manitoba in November 1974 and the Royal Victoria Hospital (RVH) in Montreal, Quebec in January 1975 (Auger, 2007; Mount, 1982). Dr. David Skelton, a British-trained geriatrician, was responsible for establishing the 'terminal care unit' in Winnipeg, while Dr. Balfour Mount, a urological cancer specialist, was responsible for establishing the palliative care programme at the RVH (Scott et al., 2016). In the early 1970s, Mount visited Dame Cicely Saunders at St. Christopher's Hospice in London, England to see for himself how the British hospice model worked. Upon his return, he created a 12-bed hospice-like unit at the RVH. Mount's palliative care programme also included a 'consultation service for people in other wards, palliative care workers who visited the dying at home, and a grief program' (Sewell, 2003, p. 89). Included among the programme's team members were trained volunteers, who provided support to patients and families in the in-patient palliative care unit, the home care outreach service, and the bereavement follow-up programmes (O'Neill, 1978).

Subsequent to these first hospital-focused palliative care programmes, 'a grassroots hospice explosion began with many of the new teams made up solely of volunteers' (Mount, 1992, p. 59). These programmes, started by dedicated groups of volunteers, were created in response to local needs. In the late 1970s, for example, a movement called the Victoria Association for the Care of the Dying was formed in Victoria, British Columbia (known today as the Victoria Hospice Society) to provide volunteer support for people who were dying in the community. By 1986, only half of the 373 hospice palliative care programmes in Canada 'were affiliated with hospitals, and of those programs that were affiliated with hospitals, 66 per cent were consulting teams, not separate hospice units' (Siebold, 1992, p. 183).

In 1988, Casey House, one of the first hospices in the world devoted exclusively to people living with HIV/AIDS opened in Toronto, Ontario (Casey House, 2016). Today, Casey House is supported by approximately 300 volunteers who, for example, provide resident support, work on reception, and raise funds for the hospice.

According to a 1990 survey of palliative care programmes in Canada, volunteers were the second most common members of palliative care teams after nurses (The Canadian Palliative Care Directory, as cited in Mount, 1992). In 1991, the Canadian Palliative Care Association (CPCA) was established, later changing its name to the Canadian Hospice Palliative Care Association (CHPCA) in recognition of 'the convergence of hospice and palliative care into one movement that has the same principles and norms of practice' (Ferris et al., 2002, p. v). The CHPCA is the national voice for hospice palliative care in Canada; its on-line directory currently lists over 600 hospice palliative care services across Canada. More complete information on the history and development of hospice palliative care in Canada is provided by Duffin (2014) and Scott et al. (2016).

Legislative and political influences

In Canada, health care is funded at both the provincial/territorial and federal levels. Under the Canada Health Act (CHA), each province and territory receives funding in support of health care from the federal government. The CHA covers hospital care and physician care. Each province and territory has other programmes (e.g. home care) that are not covered by the CHA. The 'lack of specified funding for HPC [*hospice palliative care*] under the CHA is a significant limitation of current Canadian health policy and a barrier to HPC program creation, sustainability, and accessibility' (Freeman, et al., 2013, p. 243).

In most Canadian provinces and territories, hospice palliative care is not a core health care service under provincial and territorial health care plans. As a result, end of life care in Canada is a 'variable experience' (Fowler and Hammer, 2013), 'a work in progress' (Williams, et al., 2010), or a 'patchwork of services' (Scott et al., 2016), depending on where you live. There are, for example, considerable differences in terms of what services are available depending on whether you live in a rural or remote area versus in a big city. Williams et al. (2010) describe palliative care in Canada as 'decidedly urban-centric'. Patients in rural areas often have to drive long distances or leave their own homes and move away from family and friends in order to receive better end of life care elsewhere (e.g. Robinson, et al., 2010).

One of the conclusions of a national dialogue on end of life care issues hosted by the Canadian Medical Association (2014) in partnership with *Maclean's* (a weekly news magazine) was that all Canadians, regardless of where they live, should have access to appropriate palliative care. Another conclusion was that Canada should develop comprehensive Canada-wide palliative care standards. Over the years, a number of reports on hospice palliative care in Canada have contained similar recommendations for improving access to end of life care (e.g. Carstairs, 2000, 2005, 2009, 2010; Kirby, 2002, Romanow, 2002, Quality End-of-Life Care Coalition of Canada, 2010). More recently, a report released by the Canadian Cancer Society (2016) stated that palliative care in Canada is in a 'critical condition', and that the federal, provincial, and territorial governments need to do more to guarantee access to high-quality palliative care for all Canadians.

For a more detailed discussion of health care legislative and other national initiatives that have influenced the development of hospice palliative care in Canada, see Williams et al. (2010) and Howell and Syme (2015).

End of life care settings

In Canada, dying people can choose to receive end of life care in a number of different settings. Canadians can, for example, if they have the necessary support and resources, die at home. As noted earlier, the availability of services (e.g. physicians doing home visits, hospice palliative care volunteers) depends on where people live. Even with assistance, however, dying at home requires a lot of support from family members who are comfortable dealing with their loved one's end of life care. Although the majority of Canadians say they would like to die in their own home, most die in institutions (Cairns and Ahmad, 2011). Despite a shift toward more home-based, community care in Canada, 'the services available for an individual palliative patient dying at home still vary considerably across provinces' (Scott et al., 2016, p. 25) and even between regions within provinces (Arnup, 2013).

Some Canadians will die in a nursing home or some other long-term care facility. Although a major location of death for older Canadians, most long-term care facilities do not have formalized palliative care programmes (Quality Palliative Care in Long-Term Care Alliance, 2016). As a result, when death is close at hand, it is not uncommon for residents to be transferred to a hospital for end of life care.

Another care option in Canada is a residential hospice, if there is one in the community. According to the Canadian Virtual Hospice (2016a), there are over 80 residential hospices across Canada. Ontario—Canada's most populous province—has the most residential hospices and the provincial government provides some of the operating dollars, with the rest coming from fundraising, donations, etc. Residential hospices combine a warm, home-like environment with around-the-clock medical care.

Another setting in which Canadians might die is a hospital—either in an acute care bed or in a designated multi-bed palliative care unit or room. Hospital palliative care units are typically decorated to create a home-like environment and feature a kitchen/dining area, family room, etc.

Hospice palliative care volunteers function effectively in all of the above care settings. Indeed, many hospice palliative care programmes (community-based and institutional) rely heavily on volunteers and could not offer the level of service they do without their involvement (Sevigny et al., 2010; Weeks and MacQuarrie, 2011).

The 'typical' Canadian hospice palliative care volunteer

A typical Canadian hospice palliative care volunteer is most likely:

+ Female
+ Married
+ Middle-aged or older
+ Not employed outside the home or retired
+ Has some post-secondary education
+ Reports some religious beliefs or affiliation

Volunteering in hospice palliative care is clearly a gendered activity, often thought of as 'women's work' (e.g. Auger, 2007; Weeks and MacQuarrie, 2011). Older men's and younger people's interest in becoming a hospice palliative care volunteer were examined in Canadian studies by Claxton-Oldfield et al. (2009) and Claxton-Oldfield et al. (2005). There is generally a perception among older men and younger people that this kind of volunteering is too emotionally demanding and they would not be able to handle it. In addition to males and young people, members of racial and ethnic minorities are also underrepresented among Canadian hospice palliative care volunteers (Jovanovic, 2012a).

As a rule, the first step in applying to become a hospice palliative care volunteer is to fill out a volunteer application form. Next, the volunteer coordinator will interview applicants to determine their suitability to work with dying persons and their families; applicants are also required to provide references, undergo a police/criminal record check, and sign a confidentiality agreement (Claxton-Oldfield and McCaffrey-Noviss, 2016).

Approaches to management and training

'A successful [*hospice palliative care*] volunteer program depends on strong leadership, skilled volunteer selection, training, role definition, continuing education, feedback and support' (Mount, 1992, p. 64). Hospice palliative care volunteers are typically managed by volunteer coordinators—their actual titles vary from programme to programme. The coordinators, like the volunteers, are mostly female (McKee et al., 2007; Osburn-Woolridge, 2007).

The primary management responsibilities of the coordinators generally include (depending on the care setting):

◆ Recruiting and interviewing volunteers

◆ Training volunteers

◆ Receiving referrals, meeting with patients/families to assess their needs, and assigning volunteers to patients/families; in many community-based programmes (where volunteers mostly visit in the patient's own home), coordinators will try to match volunteers with patients, taking into consideration things like age, shared interests/hobbies, etc., while in many hospital-based programmes, volunteers often work shifts and visit all of the patients on the palliative care unit who would like to be visited

◆ Making sure volunteers have all the necessary information they need to support patients/families

◆ Providing on-going support to volunteers

◆ Providing on-going training/educational opportunities for volunteers

◆ Dismissing volunteers who have overstepped boundaries (e.g. breached patient confidentiality)

◆ Providing feedback to the volunteers about their performance

◆ Keeping accurate and complete records of volunteer personnel, patient referrals, etc.

◆ Overseeing the running of the programme's office

◆ Promoting public awareness about hospice palliative care

◆ Meeting with/reporting to the board of directors

◆ Serving as a link between the volunteers and the other members of the formal caregiving team (e.g. doctors, nurses, etc.)

- Organizing memorial services
- Fundraising
- In some programmes, formally evaluating the volunteers' performance

Training

Training is critical to ensure that hospice palliative care volunteers are prepared for their role in supporting dying persons and their families. Although training programmes vary between organizations, as a general guide, the core topics that are typically covered during volunteer training include:

- The philosophy and goals of hospice palliative care
- The role of the volunteer and other members of the team
- Effective communication skills
- Family and family dynamics
- Emotional/psychological issues and support
- Spiritual/religious issues and support
- Multi-cultural issues and support
- Physical issues and support
- Caring for people at home or in a hospice
- Grief and bereavement
- Self-care

The results of a national hospice palliative care volunteer training survey revealed that all of the above topics were covered in at least 90 per cent of the 58 programmes (community- and institutional-based) that responded to the survey (Claxton-Oldfield and McCaffrey-Noviss, 2016). For more detailed information about volunteer training in Canada, see, for example, *Hospice Palliative Care Volunteers: A Training Program*, developed in 2012 by the CHPCA. This 30-hour volunteer training programme was designed with the intention of it being used across Canada to 'ensure that volunteers receive the consistent training and information they need to provide high quality of services.' That is not to say that the facilitators of volunteer training (usually the coordinators) cannot supplement their organization's training programme with resources they already have and use. Each organization has its own unique challenges and opportunities. Volunteers typically receive an orientation to the organization and its policies and procedures during training.

As a general guide, most volunteer training programmes include guest speakers (e.g. current volunteers, nurses), case studies, stories and anecdotes, handouts, films, etc. The results of Claxton-Oldfield and McCaffrey-Noviss's (2016) survey revealed that organizations offer volunteer training, on average, twice a year; half of the responding organizations pay the costs of training and just over 60 per cent require a minimum commitment of time from volunteers. The mean length of training for volunteers across programmes was approximately 28 hours. Over the years, some provinces (e.g. Nova Scotia, Ontario, British Columbia) have developed their own volunteer training manuals.

The evaluation of a training programme in New Brunswick revealed that, after training, volunteers felt significantly more able to cope with death and dying than before (Claxton-Oldfield et al., 2007). In a study by Stecho et al. (2012), Canadian medical students who participated in a pilot hospice palliative care volunteer programme (i.e. received 20 hours of training and were matched with a seasoned volunteer) had significantly lower death anxiety and communication apprehension compared to medical students who did not receive this experience.

Following training, volunteer coordinators will often have a final interview with each volunteer.

Additional training topics

In light of Canada's new medical assistance in dying (MAID) law (Bill C-14) which came into effect in mid-June 2016, I believe that hospice palliative care volunteers should be informed of their organization's stance on MAID and receive some training on how to respond in the event that a patient they are supporting wants to talk about, or access, it.

Additionally, in a recent study by Claxton-Oldfield and Dunnett (2016), 96 per cent of the Canadian hospice palliative care volunteers surveyed felt that information about unusual end of life experiences (e.g. deathbed visitations) should be included in their volunteer training. In another study by Claxton-Oldfield and Blacklock (2016), more than three-quarters of the hospice palliative care volunteers surveyed felt they needed additional training to more effectively occupy both a programme and patient/family advocate role.

Other important topics that also deserve to be included (or receive more attention) during volunteer training include supporting terminally ill patients with dementia and pediatric palliative care.

Volunteer role

Volunteers provide a broad range of supportive activities to dying persons and their families. The tasks that volunteers take on vary depending on which care setting they are volunteering in (e.g. hospital, dying person's own home, residential hospice) as well as each programme's policies and procedures. Downe-Wamboldt and Ellerton (1986), Ellerton and Downe-Wambolt (1987) and Brazil and Thomas (1995) studied the role of volunteers in hospital-based palliative care programmes in Canada. In Brazil and Thomas' (1995) study, the description of the volunteers' activities revealed that their role was primarily to provide social support. Downe-Wamboldt and Ellerton (1986) and Ellerton and Downe-Wambolt (1987) found that the volunteers' most frequently reported activities with patients and families were providing emotional support. Sevigny et al. (2010) examined the role of volunteers who provide care in patients' homes in Alberta, British Columbia, and Quebec. In this study, volunteers perceived their role in terms of, for example, developing relationships with their patients (e.g. being present), providing respite to family caregivers, providing comfort, and moral support.

As a general guide, hospice palliative care volunteers who have direct contact with patients and families can provide the following types of support (depending on the care setting):

◆ Emotional support (e.g. 'being there', providing a listening ear)

◆ Social support (e.g. friendship and companionship, sharing hobbies/ interests with the patient)

◆ Practical support (e.g. running errands for the patient/family, driving the patient to medical appointments, providing respite for the patient's family)

◆ Informational support (e.g. informing the patient/family about community programmes/resources that may be helpful to them, acting as a link between the patient/family and medical staff)

◆ Spiritual/religious support—if this is what the patient/family wants and if the volunteer is comfortable with this (e.g. praying with the patient, reading from scared writings)

Depending on the programme's policies and procedures, some programmes allow volunteers to provide personal care, for example, help with feeding, turning in bed, and getting in and out of bed. For example, in a hospital or residential hospice setting, volunteers are generally not able to provide any 'hands-on' patient care (e.g. turn patients in bed, assist with feeding), while in the private setting of a patient's home, volunteers tend to perform a broader range of activities. Some programs also have volunteers who provide various complementary therapies (e.g. music therapy, massage therapy, Reiki; see, for example, Oneschuk, et al., 2007).

As indicated above, what the volunteer can and cannot do varies across care settings. In the patient's own home, for example, where volunteers are often alone with patients, they tend to have more autonomy and flexibility than they do in, say, a hospital or residential hospice, where health care professionals are always close at hand to assist them and union rules limit what volunteers can do (Sevigny, et al., 2010). The one thing that all volunteers, regardless of the care setting, are definitely not permitted to do is prepare or administer medications to patients.

In all care settings, but especially in patients' homes, it is important that volunteers are aware of boundaries and the limits of their role (Claxton-Oldfield et al., 2011; Rothstein, 1994). As noted earlier, volunteer practices are guided by each organization's policies and procedures, which are designed to protect everyone (patients, families, and volunteers) and prevent litigation.

When a patient dies, volunteers often attend the funeral, wake, or memorial service. Some volunteers provide grief and bereavement support after a patient's death (e.g. facilitating peer support groups). Grief and bereavement support volunteers usually receive additional training, over and above the mandatory volunteer training described earlier.

To ensure the delivery of consistent, high quality visiting hospice palliative care volunteer services, Hospice Palliative Care Ontario (HPCO)—the provincial association for hospice palliative care in Ontario—has an accreditation programme for visiting hospice palliative care volunteer services. HPCO has developed standards around volunteer screening, training, scope of practice, and support and supervision. Although not required, accreditation demonstrates that the volunteer programme meets provincial standards.

Of course, volunteers can also help hospice palliative care programmes by providing non-direct patient/family support, such as administrative support (e.g. promoting awareness of hospice palliative care in the community, helping with fundraising) or working in a hospice shop (if the organization has one). In residential hospices, volunteers might also help with such tasks as gardening, reception, and so on. In most programmes, administrative volunteers do not undergo the same training that direct patient/family contact volunteers do (Claxton-Oldfield and McCaffrey-Noviss, 2016). The volunteer tasks described above are not exhaustive, but are intended to give a better idea of the many ways volunteers can support both their programmes and their patients/families across care settings.

As Mount noted in 1982, 'the best volunteers seem to have a calm and peace about them and are able to communicate this in a quiet and unobtrusive way. They must be flexible in their acceptance of different cultural and religious orientations so that they can serve patients and families without imposing their own values on others' (p. 35). For more information on the characteristics of effective volunteers, see Claxton-Oldfield and Banzen (2010).

Nurses' perceptions of the volunteer role have been examined in two Canadian studies (Downe-Wambolt and Ellerton, 1986; Claxton-Oldfield et al., 2008). Unlike the task-oriented role of nurses, volunteers have the time to just 'be there' (McKee, et al., 2010), allowing nurses to perform their tasks without having to worry about a patient being left alone. Brazil and Thomas (1995) noted that members of the hospital staff are very appreciative of the assistance provided by volunteers and a recent report by the Canadian Medical Association (2015) recommends that, in order to overcome the current challenges in palliative care, Canadian 'physicians support the valuable work of hospice volunteers' (p. vii). The positive impact of volunteers on patients and family caregivers who have utilized their service has been reported in a number of Canadian studies (e.g. Claxton-Oldfield, 2015a, 2015b; Claxton-Oldfield et al., 2010; McGill et al., 1990; Weeks et al., 2008).

Although working with dying people can be challenging, hospice pallia-tive care volunteers in Canada generally report high levels of satisfaction (e.g. Chevrier et al., 1994; Claxton-Oldfield and Claxton-Oldfield, 2012; Pascuet, et al., 2012) and often say that they feel privileged, honoured, and blessed to be able to accompany the dying and their families (Arnup, 2011; McKee et al., 2010). A couple of Canadian studies have looked at the impact of volunteering on the volunteers' lives (Claxton-Oldfield and Claxton-Oldfield, 2007; Guirguis-Younger and Grafanaki, 2008). Impacts that emerged in Guirguis-Younger and Grafanaki's (2008) interviews with volunteers included personal growth and a greater appreciation of the preciousness of life.

Changes, challenges, and successes

As Canada's population ages, the demand for quality end of life care, including the support that trained volunteers provide to dying persons and their families is likely going to increase dramatically over the coming decades. It is estimated that Canadians aged 65 years and older will make up as much as a quarter of the total population by the year 2036 (Statistics Canada, 2016). 'Therefore, the [*hospice palliative care*] field must value and nurture its volunteers; it must also assess whether the potential volunteer workforce will be large enough and have enough support to meet growing needs' (Canadian Hospice Palliative Care Association, 2009, p. 14). Some Canadian researchers have expressed con-cern about the danger of community-based volunteers' roles becoming too prescribed or task-oriented (e.g. do this and not that, stay this long), when what many volunteers really want is the freedom (or flexibility) to tailor their care for each patient (i.e. to do what is needed to best serve the patient/family they are supporting) (Guirguis-Younger, Kelley, and McKee, 2005; Guirguis-Younger and Grafanaki, 2008; McKee, Kelley, and Guirguis-Younger, 2007). It is important to not lose sight of the fact that volunteers are natural helpers and not professional helpers.

Canada is a culturally diverse society and different cultures have different expectations and needs regarding end of life care. The lack of ethnic, cultural, and linguistic diversity among hospice palliative care volunteers in the Greater Toronto Area in Ontario was identified in a study by Jovanovic (2012a), prompting her to make recommendations for more cultural competency training (Jovanovic, 2012b). The Canadian Virtual Hospice (2016b)—one of the most comprehensive websites in the world on palliative, end of life care, loss, and grief—recently launched a new website (www.livingmyculture.ca) to help health care providers (e.g. doctors, nurses, volunteers) provide more culturally safe care for people from different cultural backgrounds (e.g. First Nations, Chinese, Iranian) (2016b). Ideally, when volunteer coordinators are recruiting new volunteers, they should look at the demographics (e.g. age, gender, race, ethnicity) of the patients their programmes typically support and try to match the diversity, if any, of those patients in the volunteers they select and train. The Canadian Virtual Hospice website also offers other online tools for volunteers and volunteer coordinators in their 'For Volunteers' section.

As mentioned earlier, among the health care challenges facing Canadians living in rural and remote communities (e.g. transportation issues, difficulties recruiting and retaining health care providers) is the lack of organized volunteer programmes (McKee, Kelly, and Guirguis-Younger, 2007). To overcome the barriers to access posed by geographic location, HPCO has created an online training programme to grow the province's volunteer capacity, making hospice palliative care volunteer training accessible to volunteers across the province, including in rural and remote communities. Where volunteer support does exist in rural areas, distance is also a challenge for volunteers (e.g. one volunteer visit may take all day to complete, many volunteers are older and may not feel comfortable driving at night or be able to lift a patient) (McKee, Kelley, and Guirguis-Younger, 2007; MacLeod, Skinner, and Low, 2012). Another challenge facing some community-based volunteer programmes is the lack of referrals (see Claxton-Oldfield and Marrison-Shaw, 2014), which has resulted in some programmes shutting their doors. Lack of understanding and awareness of hospice palliative care services continues to be a big problem in Canada.

The success of Canada's volunteers has been measured not just by the impact on the volunteers themselves (Claxton-Oldfield and Claxton-Oldfield, 2007), but also on the family members of patients who have been helped by volunteers (Claxton-Oldfield, et al., 2010; Weeks, McQuarrie, and Bryanton, 2008). In both of these studies, family members indicated that they were very satisfied with the quality of support provided by volunteers. Anecdotal evidence in the form of cards and letters of thanks and appreciation from the family members also show how much they value the volunteers' help (Brazil and Thomas, 1995).

Conclusion

Across Canada, hospice palliative care volunteers provide countless hours of support to patients and families, raise vital funds to support their organizations, and make a real difference in their patients'/families' lives. Dr. Balfour Mount, who is widely regarded as the father of hospice palliative care in Canada, summed up how he (and many others) feels about Canada's hospice palliative care volunteers ... they 'are a national treasure.' (1992, p. 62).

References

Arnup, K. (2011) Caring to the end: The meanings of hospice volunteering. *Transition* **41**(1): 9–12.

Arnup, K. (2013) *Death, dying and Canadian families.* The Vanier Institute of the Family. Available from: http://vanierinstitute.ca/wp-content/uploads/2015/12/CFT_2013-11-00_EN.pdf.

Auger, J. (2007) *Social perspectives on death and dying* (second edition). Halifax, NS: Fernwood Publishing.

Brazil, K., and Thomas, D. (1995) The role of volunteers in a hospital-based palliative care service. *Journal of Palliative Care* **11**(3): 40–2.

Cairns, B., and Ahmad, M. (2011). Choosing where to die. Allowing for choices: dying at home, in a hospice or in palliative care. CBC News. Available from: http://www.cbc.ca/news/health/choosing-where-to-die-1.1002383 [Accessed 18.02.2016.]

Canadian Cancer Society (2016). Right to care: Palliative care for all Canadians. Avaialble from: https://www.cancer.ca/~/media/cancer.ca/CW/get%20involved/take%20action/Palliative-care-report-2016-EN.pdf?la=en.

Canadian Hospice Palliative Care Association (2009). Caring for Canadians at end of life: A strategic plan for Hospice, Palliative and End-of-Life Care in Canada to 2015. Available from: http://www.chpca.net/media/7562/chpca_strategic_plan_2010_2015.pdf.

Canadian Medical Association (May, 2015). *Palliative care: Canadian Medical Association's national call to action. Examples of innovative care delivery models, training opportunities and physician leaders in palliative care, 2014-2015.* Available from: https://www.cma.ca/Assets/assets-library/document/en/advocacy/palliative-care-report-online-e.pdf.

Canadian Medical Association (June, 2014). *End-of-life care: A national dialogue.* Canadian Virtual Hospice (2016a). Residential hospices. Available from: www.virtualhospice.ca/en_US/Utilities/Search.aspx?q=residential+hospices

Canadian Virtual Hospice (2016b). LivingMyCulture.ca. Available from:http://livingmyculture.ca/culture/.

Carstairs, S. (2000) *Quality end-of-life care: The right of every Canadian.* Final report of the subcommittee to update *Of Life and Death* of the standing senate committee on social affairs, science and technology. Senate of Canada.

Carstairs, S. (2005) *Still not there. Quality end-of-life care: A progress report*. Senate of Canada.

Carstairs, S. (2009) *Canada's aging population: Seizing the opportunity*. Final report of the special senate committee on aging. Senate of Canada.

Carstairs, (2010) *Raising the bar: A roadmap for the future of palliative care in Canada*. Senate of Canada.

Casey House (2016) *About Casey house ... Our history*. Available from: http://www.caseyhouse.com/about-casey-house/our-history/

Chevrier, F., Steuer, R., and MacKenzie, J. (1994) Factors affecting satisfaction among community based hospice volunteer visitors. *American Journal of Hospice Care*. **11**(4): 30–7.

Claxton-Oldfield, S. (2015a) Got volunteers? The selection, training, roles, and impact of hospice palliative care volunteers in Canada's community-based volunteer programs. *Home Health Care Management and Practice* **27**(1): 36–40.

Claxton-Oldfield, S. (2015b) Hospice palliative care volunteers: The benefits for patients, family caregivers, and the volunteers. *Palliative and Supportive Care* **13**(3): 809–13.

Claxton-Oldfield, S., and Banzen, Y. (2010) Personality characteristics of hospice palliative care volunteers: The 'Big Five' and empathy. *American Journal of Hospice and Palliative Medicine* **27**(6): 407–12.

Claxton-Oldfield, S., and Blacklock, K. (2016) Hospice palliative care volunteers as program and patient/family advocates. *American Journal of Hospice and Palliative Medicine*. Advance online publication. doi: 10.1177/1049909116659464.

Claxton-Oldfield, S., and Claxton-Oldfield, J. (2012) Should I stay or should I go?: A study of hospice palliative care volunteer satisfaction and retention. *American Journal of Hospice and Palliative Medicine* **29**(7): 525–30.

Claxton-Oldfield, S., and Claxton-Oldfield, J. (2007) The impact of volunteering in hospice palliative care. *American Journal of Hospice and Palliative Medicine* **24**(4): 259–63.

Claxton-Oldfield, S., and Dunnett, A. (2016) Hospice palliative care volunteers' experiences with unusual end-of-life phenomena. *OMEGA—Journal of Death and Dying*. Advance online publication. doi: 10.1177/0030222816666541.

Claxton-Oldfield, S., and Marrison-Shaw, H. (2014) Perceived barriers and enablers to referrals to community-based hospice palliative care volunteer programs in Canada. *American Journal of Hospice and Palliative Medicine* **31**(8): 836–44.

Claxton-Oldfield, S., and McCaffrey-Noviss, W. (2016) *Canadian Hospice Palliative Care Volunteer Training Survey (Spring 2016) Summary of Results*. Available from: http://www.chpca.net/volunteers/canadian-hospice-palliative-care-volunteer-training-survey-(spring-2016)-summary-of-results.aspx

Claxton-Oldfield, S., Crain, M., and Claxton-Oldfield, J. (2007) Death anxiety and death competency: The impact of a palliative care volunteer training program. *American Journal of Hospice and Palliative Medicine* **23**(6): 464–8.

Claxton-Oldfield, S., Gibbon, L., and Schmidt-Chamberlain, K. (2011) When to say 'Yes' and when to say 'No': Boundary issues for hospice palliative care volunteers. *American Journal of Hospice and Palliative Medicine* **28**(6): 429–34.

Claxton-Oldfield, S., Guigne, S., and Claxton-Oldfield, J. (2009) How to attract more males to community-based hospice palliative care volunteer programs. *AmericanJournal of Hospice and Palliative Medicine* **26**(6): 439–48.

Claxton-Oldfield, S., Hastings, E., and Claxton-Oldfield, J. (2008) Nurses' perceptions of hospice palliative care volunteers. *American Journal of Hospice and Palliative Medicine* **25**(3): 169–78.

Claxton-Oldfield, S., Gosselin, N., Schmidt-Chamberlain, K., and Claxton-Oldfield, J. (2010) A survey of family members' satisfaction with the services provided by hospice palliative care volunteers. *American Journal of Hospice and Palliative Medicine* **27**(3): 191–96.

Claxton-Oldfield, S., Tomes, J., Brennan, M., Fawcett, C., and Claxton-Oldfield, J. (2005) Palliative care volunteerism among college students in Canada. *American Journal of Hospice and Palliative Medicine* **22**(2): 111–18.

Downe-Wamboldt, B., and Ellerton, M. (1986) A study of the role of hospice volunteers. *The Hospice Journal* **1**(4): 17–31.

Duffin, J. (2014) Palliative care: the oldest profession? *Canadian Bulletin of Medical History* **31**(2): 205–28.

Ellerton, M., and Downe-Wamboldt, B. (1987) The concerns of hospice patients and the role of hospice volunteers *Journal of Palliative Care* **3**(1): 16–22.

Ferris, F.D., Balfour, H.M., Bowen K., Farley, J., Hardwick, M., Lamontagne, C., Lundy, M., Syme, A., West, P. (2002) *A Model to Guide Hospice Palliative Care*. Ottawa, ON: Canadian Hospice Palliative Care Association.

Fowler, R., and Hammer, M. (2013) End-of-life care in Canada. *Clinical and Investigative Medicine* **36**(3): 127–32.

Freeman, S., Heckman, G., Naus, P.J., and Marston, H.R. (2013) Breaking down barriers: Hospice palliative care as a human right in Canada. *Educational Gerontology* **39**(4): 241–9.

Guirguis-Younger, M., and Grafanaki, S. (2008) Narrative accounts of volunteers in palliative care settings. *American Journal of Hospice and Palliative Medicine* **25**(1): 16–23.

Guirguis-Younger, M., Kelley, M. L., McKee, M. (2005) Professionalization of hospice volunteer practices: What are the implications? *Palliative and Supportive Care* **3**(2): 143–4.

Hospice palliative care volunteers: A training program (2012). Available from: http://market-marche.chpca.net/Hospice-Palliative-Care-Volunteers--A-Training-Program---Printed-version

Howell, D., and Syme, A. (2015) Palliative care in Canada. In Ferrell, B., Coyle, N., Paice, J. (eds), *Oxford textbook of palliative nursing (fourth edition)*. Oxford: Oxford University Press.

Jovanovic, M. (2012a) Cultural competency and diversity among hospice palliative care volunteers. *American Journal of Hospice and Palliative Medicine* **29**(3): 165–70.

Jovanovic, M. (2012b) Improving cultural competency among hospice and palliative care volunteers: Recommendations for social policy. *American Journal of Hospice and Palliative Medicine* **29**(4): 268–78.

Kirby, M.J.L. (2002) *The health of Canadians—the federal role. Volume six: Recommendations for reform*. Final report of the standing senate subcommittee on social affairs, science and technology. Senate of Canada.

MacLeod, A., Skinner, M.W., Low, E. (2012) Supporting hospice volunteers and caregivers through community-based participatory research. *Health and Social Care in the Community* **20**(2): 190–8.

McGill, A., Wares, C., and Huchcroft, S. (1990) Patient's perceptions of a community volunteer support program. *American Journal of Hospice and Palliative Care* **7**(6): 43–5.

McKee, M., Kelley, M.L., and Guirguis-Younger, M. (2007) So no one dies alone: A study of hospice volunteering with rural seniors. *Journal of Palliative Care* **23**(3): 163–72.

McKee, M., Kelley, M.L., Guirguis-Younger, M., MacLean, M., and Nadin, S. (2010) It takes a whole community: The contribution of rural hospice volunteers to whole-person palliative care. *Journal of Palliative Care* **26**(2): 103–11.

Mount, B.M. (1992) Volunteer support services, a key component of palliative care. *Journal of Palliative Care* **8**(1): 59–64.

Mount, B.M. (1982) Palliative care of the dying. In **I. Gentles** (ed.), *Care for the dying and the bereaved*. Toronto, ON: Anglican Book Centre.

O'Neill, S. (1978) Palliative care at the Royal Victoria Hospital. *The Canadian Nurse* **74**(10): 3.

Oneschuk, D., Blaneaves, L., Verhoef, M., Boon, H., Demmer, C., and Chiu, L. (2007) The status of complimentary therapy services in Canadian palliative care settings. *Supportive Care in Cancer* **15**(8): 939–47.

Osburn-Woolridge, D.R. (2007) *Palliative care in Ontario: Hospice coordinators'experiences of providing services in small town and rural communities*. Unpublished M.A. thesis (coordinators' summary), Laurentian University.

Pascuet, E., Beauchemin, L., Vaillancourt, R., Cowin, L., Ni, A., and Rattray, M. (2012) Volunteer satisfaction and program evaluation at a pediatric hospice. *Journal of Palliative Medicine* **15**(5): 567–72.

Quality End-of-Life Care Coalition of Canada (January 2010). *Blueprint for action 2010-2020*. Available from: http://www.qelccc.ca/media/3743/blueprint_for_action_2010_to_2020_april_2010.pdf

Quality Palliative Care in Long Term Care (2016). *Long-term care homes: Hospice of the future*. Available from: http://www.palliativealliance.ca/assets/files/OLTCA_final1.pdf

Robinson, C.A., Pesut, B., and Bottorff, J.L. (2010) Issues in rural palliative care: Views from the countryside. *The Journal of Rural Health* **26**(1): 78–84.

Romanow, R.J. (2002) *Building on values: The future of health care in Canada*. Final report of the royal commission on the future of health care in Canada. Government of Canada.

Rothstein, J.E. (1994) Ethical challenges to the palliative care volunteer. *Journal of Palliative Care* **10**(3): 79–82.

Scott, J.F., Pereira, J., and Lawlor, P. (2016) Development of palliative care in Canada. In Bruera, E., Higginson, I., von Guten, C.F., and Morita, T. (eds), *Textbook of palliative medicine and supportive care* (second edition). FL: Boca Raton.

Sevigny, A, Dumont, S., Cohen, S.R., and Frappier, A. (2010) Helping them live until they die: Volunteer practices in palliative home care. *Nonprofit and Voluntary Sector Quarterly* **39**(4): 734–52.

Sewell, D. (August, 2003) Giving the gift of peace: Palliative care helps families—and their dying loved ones—cope. *Reader's Digest*, 86–91.

Siebold, C. (1992). *The hospice movement: Easing death's pains*. New York, NY: Twayne Publishers.

Statistics Canada. (2016) Population projections for Canada, provinces and territories—2009 – 2036, Catalogue 91-520-XIE. Available from: http://www.statcan.gc.ca/daily-quotidien/100526/dq100526b-eng.htm

Stecho, W., Khalaf, R., Prendergest, P., Geerlinks, A., Lingard, L., and Schulz, V. (2012) Being a hospice volunteer influenced medical students' comfort with dying and death: A pilot study. *Journal of Palliative Care* **28**(3): 149–56.

Weeks, L.E., and MacQuarrie, C. (2011) Supporting the volunteer career of male hospice palliative care volunteers. *American Journal of Hospice and Palliative Medicine* **28**(5): 342–49.

Weeks, L.E., MacQuarrie, C., and Bryanton, O. (2008) Hospice palliative care volunteers: A unique care link. *Journal of Palliative Care* **24**(2) 85–93.

Williams, A.M., Crooks, V.A., Whitfield, K., Kelley, M., Richards, J., DeMiglio, L., and Dykeman, S. (2010) Tracking the evolution of hospice care in Canada: A comparative case study analyses of seven provinces. *BMC Health Services Research* **10**: 147. Available from: https://doi.org/10.1186/1472-6963-10-147

Chapter 9

Volunteering in the United States of America

Greg Schneider

Brief history of hospice and palliative care volunteering in the United States of America

A brief comment about the term '*hospice and palliative care volunteer.*' This chapter will predominantly use the term '*hospice volunteer*' in lieu of that term. In the United States of America (USA) hospice volunteering became well established before the term palliative care began being associated with hospice care. When the term '*hospice and palliative care volunteer*' is used in this chapter, it generally refers to volunteers providing palliative care under the direction of a hospice.

How hospice began in the USA

In 1963, the British physician, Dame Cicely Saunders, initiated the introduction of the hospice concept to the USA on a lecture tour to share her work with academic and healthcare institutions. Saunders' work especially resonated with Florence Wald, then Dean of the Yale School of Nursing. Wald, a prominent proponent of social and healthcare reform, invited Saunders to return in 1966 to serve as a visiting professor at Yale and assist with the founding of the Institute on Care of the Terminally Ill. In 1968, Wald resigned as Dean and actively began to reform care for the dying by doing research studies and forming the community-based volunteer organization Hospice Inc. (now Connecticut Hospice, Inc.), the first modern hospice programme in the USA. (Buck, 2011)

In 1969, Dr Elisabeth Kübler-Ross published her seminal book *On Death and Dying*, which helped to encourage an open dialogue on the taboo topic of death and needs of the terminally ill among the general public and healthcare professionals. In addition, her book based upon years of work with the dying as well as her relentless activism on establishing better care for the terminally ill, were influential in helping federal lawmakers in Washington, DC. to begin to understand the need for better care of the dying.

The decade that followed was a time of active efforts by proponents of the hospice concept to:

◆ *Introduce Legislation*—in 1974 Congress introduced, yet did not vote upon, the first legislation to provide federal funds to support development of hospice programmes.

◆ *Establish viability of the hospice concept*—in 1978 the US Department of Health, Education, and Welfare (HEW) task force reported that 'the hospice movement as a concept for the care of the terminally ill and their families is a viable concept and one which holds out a means of providing more humane care for Americans dying of terminal illness while possibly reducing costs. As such, it is the proper subject of federal support.' This led to the financing of dozens of hospice demonstration programmes across the country.(HEW Secretary's Task Force on Hospice,1978)

◆ *Establish Hospices*—the National Cancer Institute funded the Hospice Demonstration Project, which first funded Hospice, Inc. and later dozens of other voluntary initiatives across the country that served the dying in hospitals and at home.

These activities by hospice proponents were generally successful and led to full recognition by the US government, which included the following:

◆ *Medicare Hospice Benefit (MHB) Legislation*—in 1982 Congress passed the first bill to establish hospice care as part of Medicare, the healthcare component of the social insurance programme in the US.

◆ *Accreditation, Certification and Regulation*—the new MHB law led to the establishment of accreditation agencies, certification processes and regulations to ensure that hospice would meet the established standards and quality of conventional healthcare in the US.

The MHB legislation was the most significant event in the history of hospice in the US. This law has empowered the hospice industry to grow very rapidly over the last 30 years. There were 6,100 hospice agencies operating at the end of 2014 providing services to nearly 2 million patients, of which an estimated 1.2 million of those patients received hospice services until death (National Hospice and Palliative Care Organization, 2015).

The historical role of volunteers in hospice care

Volunteers were the driving force behind the grassroots development of the hospice concept in the USA. The growing awareness of how hospitals were treating the dying inspired these individuals to come forward and begin providing the care that the hospice concept offered.

In the mid-1970s, hospice care concepts resonated with many and inspired lay people and healthcare professionals to come forward and offer their services as volunteers. Voluntary initiatives began to proliferate across the US. Three hospice care models emerged (Buck, J., 2011):

* *Hospital-based*—this model provided services with the traditional multidisciplinary teams found in hospitals. In general, lay volunteers were not part of the team.

* *Home Hospice*—nurses, commonly associated with Visiting Nurses Associations (VNAs), provided most of the medical care to patients while family caregivers attended to their common daily needs. This model involved small lay volunteer programmes.

* *Independent Hospice*—their funding came, not from government sources, but rather from foundations and charitable giving. Services were provided through collaborations with VNAs and hospitals. This model also involved lay volunteers.

The roles of volunteers have continually changed throughout the history of hospice care. The reasons for this will be discussed later. Clearly, the primary role of volunteers has been and always will be patient care. While the entire hospice team began as volunteers, the evolution of hospice and its gradual migration into mainstream healthcare has narrowed the volunteers' roles. By necessity and regulatory stipulations, paid professionals must now fulfill the majority of the roles volunteers historically filled in hospice (Connor, 2009).

Centers for Medicare and Medicaid Services (CMS) states that hospice volunteers are permitted to fill any role within the hospice, if the volunteer filling the role meets the appropriate qualifications of the *Medicare and Medicaid Programs: Hospice Conditions of Participation: Final Rule* and any other applicable State and local requirements (for example, State licensure). Since volunteers may be deployed in any role, defining specific volunteer roles is purposefully avoided by this rule. Any definition may unintentionally constrain a hospice's involvement of volunteer services, thus compromising its ability to comply with the requirements of this rule (Department of Health and Human Services, Centers for Medicare and Medicaid Services, 2008).

Administrative support volunteers—an alternative to direct patient care

'The beauty of this engagement between the volunteer and the patient is that it can transpire free of knowledge of the patient's past. No baggage needed for this journey. The trip's focus becomes each moment of life remaining.'

A Thought from the Author

It could be said that being a hospice volunteer serving dying patients is one of the most challenging, yet most rewarding, altruistic endeavors an individual could undertake. Therefore, some volunteers prefer to do administrative tasks as a volunteer as opposed to providing care to patients. This is an alternative path to becoming a direct patient care volunteer that gives the volunteer some time to first become familiar with the type of work volunteers do with patients and then to gradually begin to serve patients.

The volunteer contributions of service

In 2014, it was estimated that 430,000 volunteers provided a total of 19 million hours of service. Not all of those hours counted toward the minimum 5 per cent total of clinical hours mandated by Medicare regulations. In that year, patient care volunteers made an average of 20 visits with an average visit time of 2.3 hours.

For Medicare compliance purposes, volunteer hours fall into three categories as shown in Table 9.1.

Only categories 1 and 2 count toward Medicare's minimum 5 per cent requirement. The usage of volunteers has declined 45 per cent, as reflected by the 5 per cent metric, from 9.4 per cent in 2003 to 5.2 per cent in 2014. Coincidentally, the number of for-profit hospices increased by 44 per cent over

Table 9.1 Medicare classification of volunteer hours

Category	Name	Description	% of Total Hours in 2014
1	*Direct Patient Care*	calls, visits, and events with patients and their caregivers	61%
2	*Clinical Support*	office work that supports the direct patient care (i.e. Category 1)	20%
3	*General Support*	all other tasks that do not fit into Categories 1 and 2	19%

Source: data from Department of Health and Human Services, Centers for Medicare and Medicaid Services. *State Operations Manual, Appendix M—Guidance to Surveyors: Hospice* (Rev. 149, 10-09-15), 2015 and National Hospice and Palliative Care Organization. *NHPCO's Facts and Figures: Hospice Care in America,* Copyright © 2015 NHPCO; www.nhpco.org

the same period. This is a logical correlation given that for-profit hospices are more likely to target the minimum 5 per cent requirement.

The authentic nature of the volunteer

What motivates a half million people to volunteer each year with hospice in the USA? Many people with a desire to serve others, perhaps unknowingly, share the innate need to be in community with like-minded individuals for this purpose. When volunteers come together for volunteer meetings and share their stories, this becomes readily apparent. Those who volunteer to support people with a life-threatening illness often do so because of a personal connection to an illness or they have had a loved one of their own die under the care of hospice.

Whatever the motivation, situations that create a feeling of kinship and, ultimately a sense of community, allow one to serve others as a 'wounded warrior'. That is, one who has personally experienced the psychosocial impacts of a serious illness, cared for others with a serious illness, or have felt the devastating impact of loss, can be openly present with another who is having the same experience. There is an authenticity that the volunteer can bring to the care of the dying that cannot be taught by others or with any training method, which is so effective in strengthening the bonds of the shared experience between the volunteer, patient, and their family.

The value of volunteers

There are three different perspectives on the value of volunteers:

- The recipient of hospice and palliative care services
- The volunteer's role in serving as a member of the community
- The provider of hospice and palliative care services

The best assessment of the value of volunteers comes from those who receive their care. The fact that people give of themselves to care for others, without an expectation of remuneration, has powerful significance to those who receive the care (Connor, 1998).

An extension of this perception is the fact that the volunteer is usually a member of the community in which they serve, which can inspire more intimacy and trust. This factor can reduce communication barriers that a professional hospice worker may face and therefore the volunteers may be able to bring valuable information to the hospice team that otherwise would not be obtainable (Armstrong-Dailey and Zarbock, 2001).

Of course, providers of hospice care also recognize that volunteers provide an economic benefit as a free resource. Volunteers are on the frontlines of hospice care and essentially become hospice ambassadors, influencing the success of their organizations (Field, 2003).

Volunteer caregiving—a peer-to-peer relationship

Caregiving volunteerism in hospices is grounded in the premise that people who are facing life's most difficult challenges can improve their ability to cope with such challenges more successfully when their care includes being supported by a trained volunteer whom they regard as a peer, as opposed to someone who is acting in a professional capacity.

In this peer-to-peer relationship the patient benefits from the volunteer's life experience and the lessons learned from it. The ensuing relationship of equals puts the volunteer in a unique position of trust and understanding, which can lead to open and unrestrained communication (Garfield and Kleinmaier, 2000).

After several visits the volunteer and patient can become trusted partners in a supportive relationship in which the volunteer uses active listening skills, develops a heightened empathy for the patient and his or her situation, and assumes a largely non-judgmental stance in doing so. Service is given freely and with compassion by the volunteer and offered in such a way that both the giver and the receiver benefit.

Legislative and political influences

Since its inception, however, there has been an ongoing stream of legislative and political influences acting upon hospice volunteer programmes. Times change. Healthcare standards change. The healthcare industry, especially hospice, has been slow to be adopt technology on a large scale. The legislative influences of the last ten years have accelerated its use.

Volunteers in hospice care mandated by US Congress

The MHB ultimately led to the establishment of rules and regulations for hospice services, currently referred to as CoPs (Department of Health and Human Services, Centers for Medicare and Medicaid Services, 2008).

The CoPs related to hospice volunteers define general standards that apply to all hospice agencies that are CMS certified (see Box 9.1).

As previously mentioned these CoPs are general in nature so as not to restrict the involvement of volunteers by being too specific. The key point to be made here is that ever since the rules and regulations were first established for hospice,

Congress mandated that volunteers must be part of every hospice programme and be actively participating as part of the team at the 5 per cent minimum level or greater. They understood the importance of ensuring that the volunteer aspect of hospice care was important to preserve. There were two reasons for this:

- The care for the dying that came out of the grassroots hospice movement set a new standard and volunteers were the reason.
- Involving volunteers also provided economic benefits to the hospice related to the overall cost of care.

Medicare compliance—meeting needs of mainstream healthcare

Hospice has been under continuous scrutiny and regulations to ensure high-quality care while at the same time striving to keep its costs of care down. While Medicare does not consider volunteer services as a 'core service' of hospice, there are now very high expectations by surveyors to ensure that volunteer care plans meet the scope and frequency of patient care visits. This very high level of expectation and scrutiny is something very new for volunteer managers and it stretches the entire volunteer team. Similarly, volunteer reporting and data integration with the clinical data is now being scrutinized at levels not seen before. The fragmented methods of non-Electronic Health Record (EHR) solutions to volunteer programme data management are being targeted by surveyors to ensure data integrity.

Medicare CoP standards—volunteer qualifications and training

The CoP (§418.78) mandating volunteer training standards is further defined in the *CMS State Operations Manual (SOM)—Appendix M—Guidance to Surveyors: Hospice*. (Department of Health and Human Services, Centers for Medicare and Medicaid Services, 2015) CMS does not provide specific requirements as to what should be included in a volunteer training programme. However, SOM *Interpretive Guidelines* direct surveyors to use the following criteria (tag **L643**) for evaluating:

- 'How does the hospice supervise the volunteers? Is there evidence that all volunteers receive the supervision necessary to perform their assignments?
- Is there documentation supporting that all the volunteers have received training or orientation before being assigned to a patient/family?
- What evidence is there that the volunteers are aware of:
  - Their duties and responsibilities;

Box 9.1 § 418.78 Conditions of participation—volunteers

The hospice must use volunteers to the extent specified in paragraph (e) of this section. These volunteers must be used in defined roles and under the supervision of a designated hospice employee.

(a) **Standard: Training**. The hospice must maintain, document, and provide volunteer orientation and training that is consistent with hospice industry standards.

(b) **Standard: Role**. Volunteers must be used in day-to-day administrative and/or direct patient care roles.

(c) **Standard: Recruiting and retaining**. The hospice must document and demonstrate viable and ongoing efforts to recruit and retain volunteers.

(d) **Standard: Cost saving**. The hospice must document the cost savings achieved through the use of volunteers. Documentation must include the following:

   (1) The identification of each position that is occupied by a volunteer.

   (2) The work time spent by volunteers occupying those positions.

   (3) Estimates of the dollar costs that the hospice would have incurred if paid employees occupied the positions identified in paragraph (d) (1) of this section for the amount of time specified in paragraph (d) (2) of this section.

(e) **Standard: Level of activity**. Volunteers must provide day-to-day administrative and/or direct patient care services in an amount that, at a minimum, equals 5 per cent of the total patient care hours of all paid hospice employees and contract staff. The hospice must maintain records on the use of volunteers for patient care and administrative services, including the type of services and time worked.

Reproduced from Department of Health and Human Services, Centers for Medicare and Medicaid Services, *State Operations Manual, Appendix M—Guidance to Surveyors: Hospice* (Rev. 149, 10-09-15), L642-L647, 2015.

- The person(s) to whom they report;
- The person(s) to contact if they need assistance and instructions regarding the performance of their duties and responsibilities;
- Hospice goals, services and philosophy;

- Confidentiality and protection of the patient's and family's rights;
- Family dynamics, coping mechanisms and psychological issues surrounding terminal illness, death and bereavement;
- Procedures to be followed in an emergency, or following the death of the patient; and
- Guidance related specifically to individual responsibilities.'

Medicare care choices model—CMS demonstration project

Through the Medicare Care Choices Model (MCCM), the CMS is providing a new option for patients to receive hospice-like support services from hospice providers selected to participate in this demonstration project while concurrently receiving curative care services. Under current MHB rules, patients are required to forgo curative care services in order to receive hospice care.

MCCM hopes to achieve:

- Increased access to supportive care services provided by hospice
- Improved quality of life and patient/family satisfaction
- Updated payment systems for the Medicare and Medicaid programmes

There is a large volunteer component associated with MCCM care and therefore is increasing the size of the volunteer force. A similar two-year study in 2004 by Aetna Insurance Company that offered hospice patients 'concurrent care' (both curative and non-curative) showed a stunning 70 per cent increase in hospice enrollment with a 25 per cent reduction in the cost of hospice care. Giving people such options is clearly important and reduces their fear of using hospice.(Gawande, 2014)

Criminal background checks—financial impact to volunteer programmes

In 2012, the CMS made criminal background checks mandatory for hospice workers. The law stipulates that any volunteer serving the elderly and frail must have Level 2 background checks and fingerprinting. Before a potential patient care volunteer can receive training, the hospice must complete this check, which is about $80. This can be a major expense for the volunteer programme; and there is no guarantee that it will get a return on that investment given the potential applicant attrition rates that can arise when preparing an individual to serve the dying.

Health Insurance Portability and Accountability Act (HIPAA) of 1996

The HIPAA privacy regulations require that healthcare providers develop and follow procedures that ensure the confidentiality and security of protected health information (PHI). 'A major goal of the Privacy Rule is to assure that individuals' health information is properly protected while allowing the flow of health information needed to provide and promote high quality health care and to protect the public's health and well-being.' (OCR Privacy Brief, 2003) This is a broadly applied law that applies across all of healthcare. Each hospice sets its own policies with regard to HIPAA resulting in a variety of interpretations and applications of the law. There is an inconsistency in the application of this law to hospice volunteer programmes, often by non-legal hospice disciplines responsible for HIPAA compliance in their organizations. This situation can unintentionally perpetuate the misapplication of this law at a hospice if there is no audit procedure to review its application. This trend is a growing concern of volunteer managers.

HITECH Act—adoption of technology for increased productivity

Established under President Obama's American Recovery and Reinvestment Act of 2009, the Health Information Technology for Economic and Clinical Health Act (HITECH Act) provided a substantial financial incentive to encourage physicians, hospitals and other healthcare providers to adopt Health Information Technology (HIT). Since 2009, there has been increasing adoption of Electronic Health Record (EHR) systems for clinical use because of its efficiency, ease of access to and accuracy of patient information.

While there are many vendors offering EHR systems for hospice clinical staff, these systems do not serve the needs of most hospice volunteer programmes. This is because of the inherent development cost to the vendor with little opportunity to recoup their investment because volunteer programmes are so cost constrained.

Many hospice volunteer programmes are still using non-EHR methods that are paper-based to report patient visits. While computer technology is generally accepted and in widespread use (Wittenberg-Lyles et al., 2011), inefficiencies abound due to manual non-EHR methods for programme management such as:

◆ Excel spreadsheets to track volunteer data and patients

◆ Patient information forms that are mailed to volunteers before an assignment

◆ Paper forms are used to report patient visits, processed by mail, or reported electronically using anonymized unencrypted email

In 2008, the Hospice Volunteer Association began to address this problem using technology-minded volunteers who developed the *Patient Data Vault (PDV)*, the only fully integrated EHR system for hospice volunteer programme management and patient visit reporting that exists today. This system, which has the ability to share information with clinical EHRs, has increased the efficiencies of hospice volunteer programmes and reduced their operating costs.

Right-to-die: assisted dying and euthanasia

The topics of euthanasia and assisted dying are among the most hotly debated topics in healthcare today. Physician-assisted suicide in the United States is legal in the states of California, Oregon, Vermont, and Washington. These topics and their associated laws are controversial and unavoidable. While hospices do their best to prepare volunteers who may have patients that are leaning towards these alternatives, volunteers should receive training on how best to respond when encountering these topics and deflect them to the professional staff.

Approaches to management and training

Hospice agencies face continued pressures to reduce costs, increase efficiency, and comply with stricter regulatory requirements, while simultaneously providing optimal care and outcomes for patients and family members. The success of a hospice volunteer programme is dependent upon good managers that can instill confidence in the volunteers with comprehensive ongoing training. The ability to retain volunteers depends on a variety of factors but perhaps most important is creating a sense of community that makes the volunteers feel safe and nurtured.

The typical volunteer training programme

In 2010 a national hospice volunteer training survey was conducted by the Hospice Educators Affirming Life (HEAL) Project (Wittenberg-Lyles, Schneider and Oliver, 2010). The survey found that volunteer coordinators are principally responsible for planning and facilitating volunteer training programmes.

Paid staff are often the educational resources for the training and the volunteers are typically trained separately from other hospice staff. Volunteer training was conducted an average of 3.2 times per year, averaging 43 volunteers trained per year. A typical training programme provides 24 hours of training completed over a seven-week time span. Survey respondents ranked training curriculum topics as follows in order of importance (Box 9.2).

A 12-month minimum commitment is typically required for a volunteer to gain access to a training session. This commitment is not a Medicare requirement. It is a self-imposed restriction to maximize the cost-benefit ratio associated with training volunteers.

Hospice patients are predominantly adults. Of the 2.6 million deaths in America in 2014, approximately 42,000 (1.6 per cent) were children (NHPCO,

Box 9.2 Training topics

Communication	Boundaries
Supporting families	Family dynamics
What is hospice care?	Policies and procedures
Being present	Grief and bereavement
Volunteerism and hospice	Spiritual care
Volunteer self-care	Cultural issues
Ethics and regulations	Care for actively dying
Physiology of dying	Diseases of dying
History of hospice	Practical bedside care
Rituals in dying	Volunteer monitoring
Touch / massage	Meditation
Music / art therapy	Pediatric care

Adapted with permission from Elaine Wittenberg-Lyles et al. Results from the National Hospice Volunteer Training Survey. *Journal of Palliative Medicine*, Volume 13, Number 3, 2010, Copyright © Mary Ann Liebert, Inc.

2015). Approximately 40 per cent of hospices have a formal pediatric care programme in place and their volunteers require specialized training to serve children and their families. Not all adult volunteers are capable of being a good pediatric volunteer. There are unique needs when serving children and their families. Therefore, careful screening and evaluation is required when selecting pediatric palliative care volunteers.

Impact of training on volunteer effectiveness and retention

A thoughtful, comprehensive training programme can be an important asset in improving volunteer effectiveness and retention. The intrinsic rewards to volunteers for serving their patients well are among the most compelling motivations for continuing their volunteer work. Volunteer satisfaction is enhanced and, with the continual reinforcement of their commitment, the volunteers stay with their work far longer. Some of the barriers to volunteer retention include:

◆ *Lack of immediate availability of a training session*—this can result in the loss of a recruited volunteer who then moves on to another volunteer opportunity in another organization.

- *Lack of immediate availability of patient assignments*—this can insert a long waiting period between completion of training and first patient assignment. This can result in the volunteer losing confidence in their ability to serve or a general loss of interest.
- *Feeling underutilized and a lack of continuity in service*—good management is required to prevent the loss of volunteers because there is a long waiting period between patient assignments.

Management challenges

One of the consistently challenging aspects to hospice volunteer management is meeting the mandatory 5 per cent of all hours for patient care services provided by hospice volunteers (Wittenberg-Lyles et al., 2011). Agency characteristics such as recruitment methods, training, geographic coverage, non-patient volunteer opportunities, and the ongoing challenges of managing volunteers are prevalent barriers to meeting this federal requirement.

The general management challenges in order of declining difficulty are:

- Volunteer's busy schedules
- Communicating with volunteers
- Training/support
- Volunteer scheduling
- Volunteer retention
- Ability to recruit enough volunteers, especially in rural areas

How and why volunteering in hospice and palliative care is changing

The forces of change have been significant, as one might expect for a service that began as an unregulated grassroots movement and has slowly migrated over the last 40 years into the highly regulated environment of mainstream healthcare. The primary forces shaping volunteering have been regulations, care quality, skill requirements, liability concerns, and changing business objectives in a highly competitive environment.

Primary forces of change

The forces of change are formidable and many:

- Regulatory Requirements—Federal Fair Labor Standards Act (FLSA) and HIPAA.
- Labour laws do not allow volunteers with for profit hospices to do activities such as general office or administrative work that are not charitable in nature.

- Arbitrary interpretations of HIPAA by some hospices are reducing and limiting the kinds of services a volunteer can perform.

- Mainstream medicine—more stringent qualifications across the board. For example, a certified massage therapist could volunteer their services to a hospice without other credentials. Now conventional institutions are requiring additional certifications to do massage on hospice patients.

- Quality of care requirements are similarly forcing an expansion of volunteer roles, skills, and specialization. However, this specialization is narrowing the opportunities for lay volunteers.

- Qualifications of volunteer managers—the responsibilities of a volunteer coordinator are expanding and these positions are now requiring college degrees.

- Volunteer demographics—while there is a broadening of age diversity, additional work needs to be done to expand cultural diversity to better serve the communities-at-large.

- Business climate—for-profit companies are the dominant competitor (Figure 9.1), which is changing business strategies and objectives of non-profit companies. For-profit companies are reducing what roles volunteers can serve due to liability concerns. Volunteer inputs into the interdisciplinary team are also being curtailed.

- Technology is changing hospice care on many fronts—being able to demonstrate compliance with care plans, patient visit reporting regulations, while

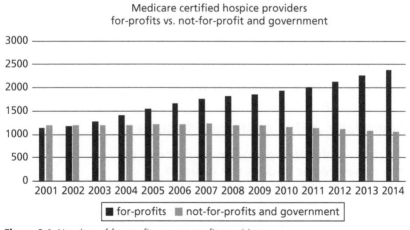

Figure 9.1 Number of for-profit vs. non-profit providers

Source: data from National Hospice and Palliative Care Organization. *NHPCO's Facts and Figures: Hospice Care in America*, Copyright © 2015 NHPCO; www.nhpco.org

maintaining HIPAA compliance are increasingly difficult if technology is not being utilized.

◆ Will the 5 per cent rule for volunteers be abolished? Some volunteer coordinators are concerned that cost pressures and desire of for-profits to maximize profits for their shareholders may lead to elimination of volunteer programmes. Surveyor's interests in volunteer-programme compliance at all levels seems to indicate this is not likely in the foreseeable future.

Primary areas of change

The areas of change due to the forces of change are both good and bad:

◆ Freedom and varieties of volunteer services offered is highly restrictive

◆ Volunteer management is multi-level as hospices get larger in size

◆ Locations where volunteer services are offered has increased

- Environment affects the volunteer experience in a variety of ways

- As variety of situations grow so do the challenges to serve

◆ Nature of new diseases such as Alzheimer's requires special training, increased specialization also requires more training

◆ Reduced diversity of roles played by volunteers in end-of-life care, making volunteering less fulfilling

◆ Stages of care broadening—broader use of palliative care, which increases the opportunities to volunteer in this discipline

◆ Specialization of volunteer roles is creating more opportunities for professionals and less for lay volunteers

◆ Misconstrued HIPAA interpretation is diminishing volunteer access to information making it more difficult to serve patients

◆ Businesses are restructuring, changing the focus of care away from the level of service traditional hospices used to provide

Some factors that contribute to success

Secret to volunteer programme success: serve the volunteer as well as the patient

The ability of an organization to recruit and retain a good volunteer force is highly dependent upon understanding that the volunteer has come to serve their organization to fulfill their own needs and desires through the service of others—not just to serve the needs of the hospice. Volunteer leaders who do not recognize this will often be unable to keep their volunteers for very long.

Create a sense of community

Regular volunteer meetings, workshops, and seminars can go a long way towards creating a sense of community. Such events give the new volunteers a chance to learn from the more seasoned volunteers. When you have a community, the volunteer programme will retain more volunteers and encourage others to join your hospice.

Improve retention—use mentoring

If you want to retain your volunteers and encourage them to grow, involve them as mentors as often as possible. Allow them to participate in the training of new volunteers. Encourage them to accompany newer volunteers on patient visits. Mentoring can be done at many levels and it will make a volunteer feel more important and more fulfilled as they see others being affected by their efforts.

Conclusions

The world of hospice and palliative care volunteerism continues to thrive in the USA. The scope and breadth of the modern day volunteer experience has diminished considerably compared to that of only a decade ago because of regulations and legal liability concerns of hospice organizations, which are now predominantly for-profit. The non-profit hospice's primary concern was solely for the patient. In these modern times, the for-profit companies have to split their concern to satisfy both the patient and their shareholders. In the end, it is the patient and their family that are impacted and indirectly the hospice and palliative care volunteer. This is not to infer that the patient is not receiving quality care, however, the care provided is different from the past.

It is possible to bring back the level of care that volunteers used to be able to provide. The reason the volunteer's role is diminishing is because the volunteer's role is not defined concretely. Medicare CoPs are intentionally vague as to roles and training required so as not to constrain how volunteers can be utilized. The downside to this is that there is not a firm definition of the volunteer's REQUIRED skills, roles and responsibilities to counter claims by lawyers that volunteers should no longer perform certain care roles with patients. Until this occurs, through the definition of agreed upon standards within the hospice community, the volunteer's role will continue to decline. This is a priority of the Hospice Volunteer Association to establish such standards and increase the volunteer's participation in patient care.

References

Armstrong-Dailey, A. and **Zarbock, S.** (2001) *Hospice Care for Children*. (1st edition). New York: Oxford University Press.

Buck, J. (2011) Policy and the reformation of hospice. *Journal of Hospice and Palliative Nursing* 13(Supplement): S35–S43.

Connor, S. (1998) *Hospice: Practice, Pitfalls, and Promise*. Washington, DC: Taylor and Francis.

Connor, S. (2009) *Hospice and Palliative Care*. 1st ed. New York: Routledge, Taylor and Francis Group.

Department of Health and Human Services, Centers for Medicare and Medicaid Services, (2008). *Federal Register, 42 CFR Part 418 Medicare and Medicaid Programs*: Hospice Conditions of Participation; Final Rule.

Department of Health and Human Services, Centers for Medicare and Medicaid Services, (2015). *State Operations Manual, Appendix M—Guidance to Surveyors*: Hospice (Rev. 149, 10-09-15). p. L643.

Department of Health, Education, and Welfare (HEW) Secretary's Task Force on Hospice. (1978). [Government Report] U.S. DEPARTMENT OF HEALTH, EDUCATION, AND WELFARE, HEW Secretary Archive. Washington DC: Available from: https://archive.org/stream/hewsecretarystas00unit/hewsecretarystas00unit_djvu.txt

Department of Health, Education, and Welfare (HEW) (1978) *Report of the Secretary's Task Force On Hospice*. [Government Report], HEW Secretary Archive. Washington DC.

Field, M. (2003) *When children die*. 1st edition. Washington, DC: National Acad. Press.

Garfield, C. and Kleinmaier, C. (2000) *Training volunteers for community service*. 1st ed. San Francisco: Jossey-Bass Publishers.National Hospice and Palliative Care Organization. NHPCO's Facts and Figures: Hospice Care in America. 2015. Available from: www.nhpco.org.

Gawande, A. (2014). *Being Mortal*. 1st edition. New York: Metropolitan Books.

OCR Privacy Brief, (2003) *Summary of the HIPAA Privacy Rule, HIPAA Compliance Assistance*. Washington DC: Department of Health, Education, and Welfare (HEW), p. 1. Available from: https://www.hhs.gov/sites/default/files/privacysummary.pdf.

Wittenberg-Lyles, E., Schneider, G. and Oliver, D. (2010) Results from the National Hospice Volunteer Training Survey. *Journal of Palliative Medicine* 13(3)261–5.

Wittenberg-Lyles, E., Shaunfield, S., Oliver, D., Demiris, G., and Schneider, G. (2011) Assessing the readiness of hospice volunteers to utilize technology. *American Journal of Hospice and Palliative Medicine* 29(6): 476–82.

Chapter 10

Volunteering in hospice and palliative care in Australia

Alex Huntir

Brief history of palliative care volunteering in Australia

Until the late 1970s and early 1980s there was little coordinated activity in palliative care. Clinicians, frustrated with poor resources for end of life care, watched modern palliative care developments abroad with increasing interest. Local palliative care initiatives started to emerge. In New South Wales (NSW) a palliative care unit was established within the Mt Carmel Surgical Hospital by 1978. In Western Australia a presentation by Cicely Saunders at a conference in 1977 gave significant impetus to the development of palliative care services (Lewis, 2006) and by 1982 the Western Australian state government had funded metropolitan-based palliative care services through a collaboration between the SilverChain nursing service and the Cancer Foundation of Western Australia (SilverChain, 2016). In South Australia Professor Ian Maddocks was instrumental in the development of palliative care services including the Southern Community Hospice Service which began operating at the Flinders Medical Centre in 1983 (Palliative Care South Australia, 2016).

A movement to establish palliative care peak bodies also gained momentum in the 1980s. Peak bodies in the Australian context are membership-based not-for-profit organizations that exist to champion and promote a cause based on systemic advocacy but without offering service delivery. These peak bodies gave collective voice to clinicians and others acting in volunteer roles to represent the emerging palliative care movement and lobby their respective state or territory government for improved resources. These efforts gave birth to what is now Palliative Care New South Wales and Palliative Care Victoria in 1981, with other states and territories to follow (Redpath, 1998). The Australian Hospice and Palliative Care Association (now Palliative Care Australia) was subsequently formed by the collective associations in 1991 to represent the needs of members to the Federal Government.

In the 1980s and 1990s there was a groundswell of community support for palliative care, and many not for profit organizations were founded in the 1980s and 1990s with an interest in community education and home support by volunteers. Some of these included the Outstretched Hand Foundation (NSW in 1980), Hospice Foundation Geelong (Victoria in 1982), Peninsula Home Hospice (Victoria in 1984), Ballarat Hospice Care (Victoria in 1985), Hospice Care Association of North West Tasmania (Tasmania in 1986), Muswellbrook Carelink (NSW in 1988), Daw House Hospice (South Australia in 1988), Ipswich Hospice Care (Queensland in 1988), Mercy Hospice (Victoria in 1990), Karuna Hospice Service (Queensland, 1992), Busselton Hospice Care (Western Australia in 1989), Byron Hospice Services (NSW in 1994), Hopewell Hospice (Queensland in 1994) and Toowoomba Hospice Association (Queensland in 1996).

The model of volunteer-intensive independent residential hospice found for example in the United Kingdom and New Zealand from the 1970s was not replicated in Australia to anywhere near the same extent, perhaps because modern palliative care was conceived as a clinical rather than a community-led initiative. In this way the local hospital networks emerged as clinical leaders in palliative care, and palliative care volunteers were supported within each local hospital network according to their facilities, resources, and local commitment. Two models of palliative care volunteer services emerged; one in which volunteers are embedded within the local hospital networks (hospitals and community health centres), and another in which volunteers are supported by an independent (typically not for profit) organization with close ties to the local hospital networks.

Palliative care volunteers can be found in all types of organizations, with variations, across different states and territories. For example, in NSW, Victoria, South Australia, and the Northern Territory palliative care volunteers are more likely to be attached to government local hospital networks than not-for-profit organizations. In Tasmania, the Australian Capital Territory, and Western Australia palliative care volunteers are more likely to be supported through not-for-profit organizations than government services.

Not all palliative care volunteering initiatives have had a long lifespan. In rural areas some palliative care volunteer services, established with or by local community nurses, proved to be vulnerable to the ebb and flow of support within the team as staff left and new staff joined (Huntir, 2016). Some services did not survive, but volunteering in rural areas tends to be higher per capita than in metropolitan and other settings, indicating that the loss of services is a feature of resourcing rather than community spirit.

Not all palliative care volunteering has been led from within the boundaries of the health system. During the 1980s and 1990s the HIV/AIDS epidemic resulted in considerable stigma against the gay community. Individuals supportive of the gay community, both inside and outside the health care system as well as within not-for-profit AIDS organizations, stepped forward as volunteers to provide in-home end of life care (Kennedy, 2016). With an increasing interest in informal networks of care these initiatives are attracting more attention for their contribution to social capital and community capacity building.

Palliative care volunteers in Australia act largely in a complementary role to assist expert palliative care clinicians and enhance end of life care in inpatient and community settings.

Typical roles undertaken by palliative care volunteers include inpatient support, community visiting (including carer respite in the home), distributing and collecting equipment, assisting with memorial services, within biography and diversional therapy programmes, as well as by performing bereavement follow up. Volunteers in paediatric settings are generally focussed on family and sibling support but they may also help parents with domestic duties, and in inpatient settings they may provide administration support, reception services, fundraising, and grounds maintenance.

Compared to other western nations, support for palliative care volunteers in Australia seems unspectacular. It is estimated that there are about 6,000 palliative care volunteers in Australia within a national population of about 24 million people (Australian Bureau of Statistics, 2014). The relatively low numbers of palliative care volunteers (by western standards) is one of the challenges in improving the legitimacy of palliative care volunteers in Australia.

In Australia there is no coordinated national effort to represent or champion palliative care volunteering, no enduring attempt to network palliative care volunteer services, nor any central repository of information or analysis about the role or contribution of palliative care volunteers. The relative obscurity of volunteers is symptomatic of the dominance of professionalization narratives in palliative and end of life care, but it also reflects the way that modern palliative care evolved in Australia.

Legislative and political influences

At a national level there are no specific legislative or strategic frameworks affecting palliative care volunteers. Systemic development of palliative care volunteers has tended to focus on volunteer services through volunteer standards, training, and capacity enhancement. For example in Victoria in 2007, the Palliative Care Volunteer Standards were published as an initiative by the state government aimed at strengthening volunteer services (Department of Human Services, 2007). In NSW in 2014, the Volunteer Support Services Programme, a state government initiative was launched with the aim of improving the support for and performance of palliative care volunteer services, with a particular interest in increasing the capacity for community-visiting roles (NSW Health, 2016).

Community hospice represents a small and unique sector providing respite and end of life care. Not-for-profit residential hospices operate in NSW, Queensland, Western Australia, and Victoria, often with higher than average volunteer involvement per service (Hansen and Huntir, 2014). Support from their respective state governments for hospice is mixed, with some hospices receiving recurrent government funding and others relying solely on fundraising. Queensland has three residential hospices in the south-eastern area of the state, and a recent state parliamentary report endorsed their model and recommended an increase in capacity (Queensland Parliament, 2013). There are also three dedicated children's hospices located in NSW, Victoria, and Queensland and each works closely with local specialist children's hospitals. In NSW it is estimated that volunteers within children's palliative care (hospitals and hospices) account for about 10–15 per cent of all palliative care volunteers in the state (Hansen and Huntir, 2014). Although there is insufficient data for comparison the experience of paediatric palliative care volunteers in NSW appears to be characterized by high levels of engagement and collegiality (Burke, 2016).

Residential aged care in Australia also functions substantially as a form of residential hospice (Queensland Parliament, 2013). Volunteers in residential aged care may participate in palliative care, although the number of volunteers in residential aged care, the number of services supporting volunteers, or the extent of their training in palliative care is unclear. The federally-funded 'Community Visitors Scheme' is a volunteer program that connects aged residents with volunteer visitors, albeit with a focus on social support rather than palliation. A pilot study in NSW in 2015 found that about 42 per cent of facilities engaged volunteers in roles which they believed represented palliative care, but that some 25 per cent of facilities had no volunteers (Burke, 2015). A lack of staff capacity to support volunteers was one reason for not hosting volunteers but different understandings of palliative care were also noted. A trial programme through Palliative Care Australian Capital Territory shared hospice volunteers with residential aged care facilities and successfully demonstrated the possibility of more creative solutions to volunteer support for people in aged care (Palliative Care Australian Capital Territory, 2016).

The challenges facing palliative care services in Australia in turn affect their volunteers. A lack of understanding of palliative care, or a reluctance to refer to palliative care, by other clinicians hampers involvement of the palliative care team at end of life. This is exacerbated by a cultural reluctance amongst individuals and families to acknowledge end of life and to request access to palliative care. Consequently referrals to palliative care are sometimes made too late to provide any meaningful support. These factors impact the degree to which volunteers can be engaged, and less engagement can result in greater obscurity within the delivery of palliative care.

Another of the challenges facing palliative care is posed by the national system which delivers funding to the local hospital networks. With the exception of aged care and services by general practitioners, Australia's federated structure largely devolves responsibility for hospital and health care service delivery to the six state and two self-governed territory governments. Funding for palliative care flows from the Federal Government to the local hospital networks within the states and territories. The contemporary Activity Based Funding model rewards local hospital networks for the efficient delivery of services by measuring clinician interventions and episodes of care. The local hospital networks are responsible for service planning within their geographic catchments, largely through clinicians working within and from public health care sites (including hospitals, community health centres, and multipurpose health services). Palliative care volunteers work with clinicians but are regarded as non-clinical. As a consequence the local hospital networks struggle to claim 'billable' services under the Activity Based Funding model for their volunteer-related activity, so the necessary funding for palliative care volunteer support must usually be found from within the resources of the local hospital network. Consequently, the level of commitment to palliative care volunteers may vary between different networks and between different sites within a network.

Mixed messages exist about the specific nature of the value of palliative care volunteers to health services. In NSW a study of promotional material identified key themes about palliative care volunteers. In some services the palliative care volunteers were championed as an additional workforce element to enhance service delivery, while in others the volunteer service was presented as a demonstration of the local hospital network's commitment to community partnerships, or of their commitment to compassionate care (Flood and Huntir, 2016).

At a state and territory level, central coordination and resourcing of palliative care volunteer services across local hospital networks is not consistent. For example in South Australia volunteer services are managed centrally within each of three regions (Northern, Central, and Southern). By comparison, in NSW the volunteer services are located within 15 health districts (eight metropolitan and seven regional), with volunteers also active within some paediatric and statewide services, but unlike South Australia, there is no centralized coordination of volunteer services within each health district.

Although service planners in local hospital networks are very supportive of the work of palliative care volunteers (Flood and Huntir, 2016) planners do not always have influence over governance arrangements or funding decisions. Consequently, expressions of support do not always translate into budget commitment by the health service. In a budget-stressed and output-focused health environment the necessary funding for non-clinical roles like palliative care volunteers is typically hard-fought for and under pressure.

The state and territory peak bodies play various roles in championing the palliative care volunteer sector. Palliative Care Australian Capital Territory is funded to host and support volunteers in the Canberra catchment, and both Palliative Care New South Wales and Palliative Care Victoria play roles in networking managers of palliative care volunteer services. Consistent commitment to networking and promotion at a national level is yet to be achieved but would do much to raise the profile of palliative care volunteering in Australia.

Approaches to management and training

In broad terms the aims of a palliative care volunteer service is to affirm the compassionate and dignity-promoting philosophy of palliative care, to offer support to people and their loved ones who have been referred to palliative care and to support the local palliative care team in delivering services to the community.

Palliative care volunteers come from all walks of life, including retired clinicians from end of life or other health settings, as well as others from business, law, or trades, and students (such as medicine, nursing, law) who undertake volunteering as an activity in addition to their study requirements. The size of the organization is proportional to the financial capacity to support the management and activities of volunteers, evidenced by more hours of work per week for volunteer managers and, on-average, higher numbers of volunteers. Table 10.1 compares observations in New South Wales for different settings (Hansen and Huntir, 2014).

Volunteer managers working in unpaid roles are more likely to be found in not-for-profit organizations, which in turn are more likely to be found in rural areas. Not-for-profit organizations and rural communities face other challenges. Smaller communities typically have less inpatient options, so palliative care volunteers are more likely to perform community visiting than inpatient support roles. As community visiting roles are relatively more intensive for the volunteer manager to oversee, their capacity to support volunteers is reduced, and this partly explains the lower numbers in not-for-profit organizations.

Table 10.1 Summary of palliative care volunteer service features in NSW 2014

	Hospital	Community health centre	Not-for-profit organization
Proportion of all volunteers in NSW[1]	70%	4%	26%
Average volunteer manager role as proportion of fulltime[2]	0.66	0.15	0.60
Volunteers per volunteer manager (average)	37	NA[3]	30
Number of services with unpaid volunteer managers	1	2	5
Number of services in Metro/ Regional areas [4]	M=15 R=8	M=0 R=4	M=1 R=10
Total number of services in NSW	23	4	11

Notes: (1) Total number of volunteers = 1,242. (2) Also known as 'fulltime equivalent'. (3) Data not comparable due to small numbers and mixed activities. (4) Refers to Metro and Regional Local Health Districts but includes paediatric services.

Source: data from Hansen L and Huntir A. *A Snapshot of Palliative Care Volunteering in NSW 2014*, Palliative Care NSW, Surry Hills, Australia, Copyright © Palliative Care NSW Incorporated, 2014.

A volunteer manager in a metropolitan service may face very different challenges, including effectively servicing the breadth and density of their catchment, meeting the needs of culturally and linguistically diverse communities, and providing coverage across the different activities of volunteers (including inpatient, community visiting, and other tasks). Whereas palliative care volunteers in regional and rural areas may undertake a diverse range of roles, some of these roles (for example, a biography service) might in a metropolitan area be regarded as more specialized and be delivered by a different volunteer group (such as by the Social Work team or the Pastoral Care team).

There are no common national performance standards to which volunteer services must comply, although many services located within local hospital networks come under the accreditation process and policy framework for their facility. Nationally, Volunteering Australia publishes the National Standards for Volunteer Involvement as a guide to assessing organizational perform-ance (Volunteering Australia, 2015), and Palliative Care Australia publishes the National Palliative Care Standards (the Standards for Providing Palliative Care for All Australians) (Palliative Care Australia, 2005) as a guide for pallia-tive care service delivery. Perhaps better known and more extensively used are the Palliative Care Volunteer Engagement Standards (Department of Human Services, 2007), a Victorian state government initiative that includes guidance on organizational as well as volunteer performance.

Typically, each palliative care volunteer service recruits and trains their volunteers. A popular training resource is published by Palliative Care Victoria, the Palliative Care Volunteer Training Resource Kit 2012 (Palliative Care Victoria, 2012), which provides volunteer managers with a starting point for the content and scope of material in a training programme. In 2015 Palliative Care NSW developed Palliare: A Handbook for Palliative Care Volunteers (Huntir, 2015) based on the Volunteer Training Resource Kit as a learning resource for volunteers. Successful completion of palliative care volunteer training is usually based on attendance, rather than on formal measures of skill or competence. Training programs can last from between two to eight days depending on the service and the diversity of their programmes. For most services the training programme plays an important role in identifying candidates unsuited to the role, and in some cases a multi-stage approach is used to shortlist, meet with each volunteer, then review their demonstrated skills and understanding of the role before they commence.

Palliative care volunteer services typically have a good reputation for the training and support of their volunteers. Nevertheless, managers often report overload resulting from managing a high number of volunteers, as well as managing often complex and late referrals and having positions which require their time to be split with other duties (nursing, fundraising, social supports coordination). In 2003 Palliative Care Australia published a Planning Guide for Services (Palliative Care Australia, 2003) which suggested a ratio of one volunteer coordinator for every 40 community volunteers, or for every 50 inpatient volunteers. While no Australia-wide figures are available, in NSW reports indicate an average of one volunteer manager to 56.4 volunteers. Smaller not-for-profit organizations support about 75 per cent of the number of volunteers found in larger organizations (41.3 volunteers per volunteer manager) mostly due to the effort of attending to other roles that impinge on the workload of the volunteer manager (Hansen and Huntir, 2014). In NSW a high turnover in volunteer manager positions has been observed with annual vacancies in the order of 33 per cent of all positions (Hansen and Huntir, 2014). It is reasonable to assume that this turnover impacts negatively on the confidence of referring clinicians, and addressing this statistic is one of the future challenges facing palliative care volunteering.

Why and how volunteering in this field is changing

Australian statistics show that participation in volunteering generally is changing with fewer people participating in volunteering (Australian Bureau of Statistics, 2014) and an increasingly selective public looking for more meaningful content and connection through their volunteering activity (Volunteering Australia, 2007). Although this suggests a reduction in the available pool of good-quality or long-term candidates this often appears not to be the case for palliative care volunteer services, with many services reporting sufficient candidates for volunteering, volunteer services with waitlists for volunteer training without having advertised, and candidates from across the lifespan well engaged in their roles.

However, those palliative care volunteer services that experience frustration in receiving referrals find volunteer retention challenging. If referrals are delayed so that there is too little time for the volunteer to form relationships with the individual and their family then the potential contribution of the volunteer service tends to be minimalized in the eyes of referring clinicians, further impeding the flow of referrals. These conditions simultaneously reduce the availability of rewarding opportunities and the longevity of volunteers.

Overly vigorous risk management and boundaries of practice by governance and management can negatively impact on the satisfaction experienced by volunteers. Frustrations are sometimes revealed in volunteer comments about what they 'can and can't do' and impinge on the satisfaction derived from their relationship with the patient and family. Examples include: whether or not a volunteer can be left alone with a young person without a parent in attendance; whether or not a service will accept the risk involved in allowing volunteers to visit people in the community; or whether or not a service will permit a volunteer to drive a patient in their own vehicle, or leave their private contact details with a patient. Some volunteers have found these restrictions too onerous, and have looked for other ways to be involved in end of life support such as through pursing training in the emerging practices of the death doula and death midwife (Hansen and Huntir, 2014).

A revival of interest in community hospice is seeing larger numbers of people volunteering in support of local independent residential facilities for end of life care. In NSW the organization operating the community hospice Wedgetail Retreat in Dulguigan represents one of the larger palliative care volunteer groups in the state (Hansen and Huntir, 2014) despite having a small local catchment and an unpaid volunteer manager. The Southern Highlands Community Hospice group in Bowral, despite having faced long challenges with planning approval for their hospice, already has some 250 volunteers raising money through local op-shops. Perhaps community hospice attracts a higher number of volunteers because it represents a closer alignment with community values, individual autonomy, and compassion; more in keeping with traditional volunteering values and less aligned with the managerial narratives of risk management.

Other new initiatives demonstrate the continued community interest in improved palliative care and provide the basis for new and innovative volunteering. Some of these include: a collaborative venture in Parkes NSW between volunteers at the local community centre, and local palliative care clinicians started in 2013; the commencement of a volunteer-led hospice-at-home programme in Warrnambool Victoria in 2015; and the colocation of the not for profit Albany Community Hospice on the grounds of the Albany Health Campus in Western Australia in 2016.

Factors that contribute to success

Three features are highlighted in this section in recognition of their significance to the success of palliative care volunteer services: support from management, skills of the volunteer manager, and acknowledging volunteers by inclusion (quotes from Hansen and Huntir, 2014).

Support from management

Some (volunteer coordinators) are supported better than others, some supervisors are more supportive than others, some services are more engaged than others... (in other places) volunteers are just another service, no- one takes any notice of it (volunteering), it's an afterthought' (Clinician, regional service, p. 16).

Struggling palliative care volunteer services are characterized by systemic problems like vague connections to clinical governance, disparate allocation of resources, a scarcity of hours for volunteer management, or the obscurity of the role of the volunteers within the service's model of care. If clinicians lack confidence in the volunteer service then their referrals to volunteers slow or cease.

A successful service will understand the inter-relatedness of: the clinical reputation of the health service; the support for the health service within the community, and the capacity of the service to attract and retain volunteers. Typically successful services enjoy a high level of organizational support both within the clinical and governance teams, indicating that the volunteers are well supported not only by their volunteer manager but also by the system.

Skills of the volunteer manager

Within the hospital system when you go into a ward it seems like everyone is so busy with their own jobs that it's hard to get staff to recognise (and acknowledge) volunteers, I understand it's busy, but that's one of the most difficult challenges' (Volunteer Coordinator, metropolitan, p. 25).

In a system within which volunteers are characterized as 'assistants to experts' rather than experts in their own right, much depends on the ability of the volunteer manager to build relationships with clinicians and win their confidence in the volunteers so as to ensure the continued flow of referrals. This is most vividly illustrated where relationships between service and clinicians have broken down and as a consequence referrals have suffered.

Nevertheless, relationship breakdown is also a systemic issue. Some services rely too heavily on the volunteer manager to represent the cause and even the aesthetic of volunteering, relegating them to tirelessly advocate for their volunteers to be included in service delivery opportunities. Unsurprisingly this can be exhausting for the volunteer manager, and may well contribute to the high turnover of volunteer manager positions referred to previously. Management support to 'get it right' is not only important in making the service work, but also in presenting the local hospital network to the community in a positive light. In some instances, commentators noted that flawed support for a fledgling volunteer service could have been a public relations disaster for the palliative care service (Huntir, 2016).

Within many services, winning and maintaining the support of the clinical and governance teams is a significant part of the volunteer manager's role, and much of the success of any particular volunteer service is attributed to the skills of the volunteer manager.

Acknowledging volunteers by inclusion

I really want to develop relationships with people at end of life, that's my passion, direct support for people around end of life...I'm time poor, so for every hour I spend time in volunteering then my business misses out, so (the nature of the volunteering) has to hold my interest'(Volunteer, p. 25).

This comment challenges one of the common beliefs about palliative care volunteers: that they are time rich and retirement aged. In reality Australian palliative care volunteers are diverse in their life experience, qualifications, age, and motivations, in particular as revealed through studies of paediatric palliative care volunteers in NSW, in which the norm is a part or full time worker (Burke, 2016). Diversity and expertise within the volunteer group benefits clients who receive services, but it can challenge the services in how they acknowledge and include volunteers. A common trap is for the governance or management to unwittingly adopt a patronizing or tokenistic approach to volunteers. Not only does this imperil the confidence with which volunteers are regarded by referring clinicians, but it can also frame the volunteer as a passive recipient of support rather than as an actively contributing co-worker in palliative care. Disenfranchized volunteers may leave, or they may stay but with low levels of engagement or actualization.

The simple goal of volunteer support must be to improve palliative care through volunteering and this is best achieved by optimizing the engagement of the volunteers. A successful palliative care volunteer service acknowledged volunteers by including them in tasks compatible with their skills. This includes roles in team leadership, recruitment and interviewing, mentoring, delivering and reviewing training material, and delivering in-service training within the volunteer service.

In summary the palliative care volunteer service must have active support through clinical and governance teams, a skilled volunteer manager, as well as a commitment to inclusive systems of management.

Conclusion

In many ways palliative care volunteer management in Australia suffers from the privileging of experts in palliative care that tends to minimize the volunteer contribution. Recent developments and examples of successful services indicate solid support for the place of the volunteer contribution in palliative care, but in many ways agreement is yet to be reached over the significance of that place and over the normalizing of the role of volunteers within the palliative care team.

With the increasing demands on the palliative care system from an aging population, and given the patchwork of state and territory approaches to the support of volunteers, there is greater need than ever for active engagement at a national level to champion and assert the value of volunteers within the Australian palliative care system.

Acknowledgements

Text extracts from Hansen, L. and Huntir, A. *A Snapshot of Palliative Care Volunteering in NSW 2014.* Palliative Care NSW, Surry Hills, Australia. Copyright © NSW Health 2014. Reproduced with permission of NSW Health. Available at: http://volunteerhub.com.au/volunteer-support-services/a-snapshot-of-palliative-care-volunteering-in-nsw-2014/ .

References

Australian Bureau of Statistics (ABS) (2014) 4159.0—*General Social Survey: Summary Results, Australia.* Canberra: ABS.

Burke, M. (2015) *Palliative Care Volunteering in Residential Aged Care Facilities in NSW: A sample study in Western Sydney LHD.* Surry Hills: Palliative Care NSW.

Burke, M. (2016) *Paediatric Palliative Care: A survey of a hospice volunteer service.* Surry Hills: Palliative Care NSW.

Department of Human Services (DHS) Victoria (2007) *Strengthening palliative care: Palliative care volunteer standards,* Melbourne: DHS.

Flood, J. and Huntir, A. (2016) *Where-to with our volunteers? Results of a survey of Palliative Care Service Development Officers in NSW.* NSW, Surry Hills: Palliative Care NSW.

Hansen, L. and Huntir, A. (2014) *A Snapshot of Palliative Care Volunteering in NSW 2014.* Surry Hills: Palliative Care NSW.

Huntir, A. (2015) *Palliare: A Handbook for Palliative Care Volunteers in NSW.* Surry Hills: Palliative Care NSW.

Huntir, A. (2016) *Faded away: The life and death of a district volunteer initiative in the bush and lessons for the future of palliative care volunteering,* Surry Hills: Palliative Care NSW.

Kennedy, M. (2016, July) *Responding to a crisis: The community response that enabled the home deaths of people living with HIV/AIDS between 1985 and 1997.* Melbourne, Vic: Paper presented at the Palliative Care Victoria Conference.

Lewis, M.J. (2006) *Medicine and Care of the Dying.* Oxford: Oxford University Press.

NSW Health, Palliative care volunteer support services. Available from: http://www.health. nsw.gov.au/palliativecare/Pages/Palliative-care-volunteer-support-services.aspx. [Accessed 05.05.2016.]

Palliative Care Australia (PCA) (2003) *Palliative Care Service Provision in Australia: A Planning Guide.* Canberra: PCA.

Palliative Care Australia (PCA) (2005) *The Standards for Providing Palliative Care for All Australians.* Canberra: PCA.

Palliative Care Australian Capital Territory (PCACT). *Aged Care Facility-based Services.* Available from: http://www.pallcareact.org.au/index.php/services/aged-care-facility-based-services. [Accessed 05.05.2016.]

Palliative Care South Australia (PCSA). *Palliative Care in South Australia.* Available from: http://www.pallcare.asn.au/about/history-of-palliative-care/palliative-care-in-south-australia. [Accessed 26.04.2016.]

Palliative Care Victoria (PCV) (2012) *Palliative Care Volunteer Training Resource Kit 2012.* Melbourne: PCV.

Queensland Parliament (2013), *Palliative and community care in Queensland: toward person-centred care.* Health and Community Services Committee, Report No. 22, May 2013.

Redpath, R. (1998) Palliative Care in Australia. In: Ramadge J. (ed.) *Australian Nursing Practice and Palliative Care: Its Origins, Evolution and Future* (Professional Development Series No. 9), pp. 1–16. Canberra: RCNA.

SilverChain, Our History. Available from: https://www.silverchain.org.au/wa/about-us/our-history. [Accessed 26.04.2016.]

Volunteering Australia (2007) *A Toolkit for Training Volunteers (Part B).* Melbourne: Volunteering Australia.

Volunteering Australia (2015) *National Standards for Volunteer Involvement.* Canberra: Volunteering Australia.

Chapter 11

Volunteering in hospice and palliative care in Africa

Fatia Kiyange

Introduction

The 67th World Health Assembly (WHA) resolution on strengthening palliative care recognizes the role of volunteers in the provision of hospice and palliative care services (WHA, 2014). Volunteers are integral to hospice and palliative care interdisciplinary teams: while in the community, volunteers delivering palliative care are central to the engagement of communities in health matters, which is a key recommendation of the World Health Organization (WHO, 2008). Volunteers also increase community awareness of palliative care building on existing African culture where *Ubuntu* means caring for each other, derived from human kindness and compassion (Kiyange F. In Radbruch et al., 2014).

Morbidity and mortality rates due to both infectious and non-communicable diseases are high in Africa. Globally, 40 million people need palliative care annually and 80 per cent of these live in low- or middle-income countries, while for children the figure is 98 per cent and almost half of them living in Africa (WHO, 2015). Caring for the 2.5 million people who die each year from human immunodeficiency virus (HIV) in sub-Saharan African countries has triggered renewed interest in voluntary-based community health programmes (Topp et al., 2015), while care is also needed for the more than 0.5 million who die from cancer (WHO, 2001, 2002). Sepulveda and Habiyambare et al., (2003), note that it is unrealistic to expect formal health service institutions, such as hospitals and clinics, to be able to provide palliative care at the community or home level. They anticipated that family members, supported by home and community-based organizations, will provide most of the care with emphasis given to home-based palliative care provided by trained family and community caregivers to counteract the severe shortage of professional healthcare workers.

This chapter examines volunteering within hospice and palliative care services in Africa elaborating on its nature, approaches and models used in the provision of hospice and palliative care. It also describes the changing nature of the work of volunteers, issues of legislation, and the volunteer role within multi-disciplinary teams. Country approaches, experiences, and models of volunteering in hospice and palliative care in Africa do vary, and useful lessons can be learnt from these variations. Important to note is that hospice and palliative care are relatively new in Africa and only a few countries have developed comprehensive services.

Perceptions, models, and role of volunteers in hospice and palliative care in Africa

A recent study in Africa showed a wide range of volunteering in palliative care (Loth et al., 2015). Most programmes for volunteers in health in sub-Saharan African countries emerged out of the need to support HIV treatment, TB treatment, and deliver services to children orphaned through HIV (Topp et al., 2015). In South Africa for example, the HIV epidemic and the overburdened public health system in the late 1990s and early 2000s spurred an increase in community caregiving (Caregivers Action Network, 2013, p. 5).

Palliative care is best delivered by a multidisciplinary team that includes doctors, nurses, community health workers, and volunteers (WHO, 2016, p. 18). The terminology for volunteers in hospice, palliative, and other health care varies across African countries, for example: community health workers (CHWs); community-based workers (CBWs); community care workers (CCWs), and community-based volunteers (CBVs) are all used. Likewise, models of volunteering vary within and between countries. CHWs differ both within and across countries, in terms of their recruitment, training, supervision, type and amount of work, and form of remuneration (Lehmann and Saunders, 2007; George et al., 2012). According to Akintola, Hlengwa, and Dageid (2013), volunteering and volunteerism have been defined in various ways but are typically understood to mean the devotion of energy and time to an activity or service without the expectation of financial reward. CHWs, according to the WHO, are members of, selected by, and answerable to the communities where they work; supported by the health system; and receive less training than formally trained health workers (Lehmann and Saunders, 2007). A community care provider, which is a term used commonly in palliative care, is someone providing care for the patient and their family, with supervision from professional care providers, but who does not have a professional qualification recognized by the Ministry of Health, for example: community health workers, community volunteers, and lay care givers. They will, however, have had some training to prepare them for their role (African Palliative Care Association, 2011).

Volunteering models can also be categorized according to the setting of the operation, or even the disease condition or intervention they support. Community-based volunteers can operate from within their communities linking with hospice and palliative care facilities, while site-specific volunteers may operate from hospice and palliative care sites. Some volunteers are tuberculosis (TB)- or antiretroviral therapy (ART)-adherence supporters, while others cover a wider range of health issues in their work based on a number of households allocated by the facilitating agency. TB- or ART-adherence supporters are patient-nominated treatment supporters who help with treatment while also providing emotional, instrumental, and material support (Duwell et al., 2013).

Volunteers can also be termed 'professional volunteers' when they are people with professional qualifications and skills which they offer through volunteering, for example a retired nurse providing services to patients without expecting any pay. Non-professional volunteers are those without professional qualifications. To add to complexity, in some countries there are government-led volunteer programmes as well as nongovernmental organization (NGO)-led programmes, operating in parallel to each other (Kiyange, 2014).

One four-country (Kenya, Lesotho, South Africa, and Uganda) action-research project managed by Khanya—African Institute for Community Driven Development (Khanya-aicdd) between 2004 and 2007, termed volunteers community-based workers and defined this as people from the community in which they live, trained for specific tasks delivered at community level, supported and supervised by a volunteer coordinator. This may be in either an NGO or government entity. (Khanya—African Institute for Community Driven Development, 2007). The research found that in, South Africa, there are both unpaid volunteers working between four and 20 hours per week as well as those paid a stipend working for 20 to 40 hours. (Khanya—African Institute for Community Driven Development, 2007). The research further highlighted that community ownership and project success was enhanced where CBWs were selected from *and by* communities they serve.

Another term for volunteers in South Africa is community care workers from a model pioneered in palliative care where they now provide the backbone of South Africa's integrated community-based home care (WHO, 2016, p. 18). Trained and supervised by a professional nurse and backed by a strong network of community organizations including the local clinic and district hospital, they help empower family members and neighbours to cope with supportive care for patients at home, relieving the health system of the burden of care. The model was initially developed by South Coast Hospice in response to the AIDS epidemic and has been refined to cater for people with other diagnoses requiring palliative care.

Volunteers benefit care services by taking on a significant work load as well as being close to the patients (Loth et al., 2015). The action research project Khanya-aicdd found both patients and family members cited CBWs as indispensible and integral to government health systems in providing human caring, health awareness, enhanced adherence to critical medicinal dosages, Directly Observed Therapy (DOT) for TB patients, and home-based care for bed-ridden patients (Khanya-aicdd, 2007; Kiyange, 2014). The same research highlighted that, in Zambia, severe human, financial, and material resource shortages and a high-HIV burden lead to HIV volunteer caregiver programmes aimed at supplementing psycho-social, material, and/or clinical support. Volunteer roles include direct patient assistance, providing psychosocial support, spiritual support, and assisting patients' families (Loth et al., 2015). Volunteers identify patients, assess them for palliative care-related concerns and symptoms, and make appropriate referrals for patients and their families to access services, as well as providing basic health and hygiene support and sometimes accompanying patients to health facilities (Kiyange, 2014). Client visitation especially for orphans and other vulnerable children (OVC) and people living with HIV (PLHIV) is another key role for volunteers in hospice and palliative care (Topp et al., 2015).

Caregivers' roles have tended to shift in response to the epidemiological changes of the HIV epidemic, as well as to the ways in which funding has prioritized the pandemic over other illnesses. In South Africa this shift is to basic physical care and other support required by clients and their families within the home environment as the HIV epidemic worsened during the 1990s. After 2004 when ART became more available, roles diversified and specialised in testing, counselling, and monitoring adherence to medication, in addition to services already provided such as psychosocial support, care for OVC, and socioeconomic support for those infected with and affected by HIV. Recent policy moves by the National Department of Health have been towards a more generalist community health worker primarily playing a surveillance and health promotion role in communities, mapping health conditions, and advising and referring the at-risk to appropriate care, support, and treatment. On the whole there is a trend towards the integration of conditions other than HIV/ acquired imunodefficiency syndrome (AIDS), most notably the integration of HIV and TB services (Caregivers Action Network, 2013).

Hospice Africa Uganda have developed a community volunteer programme, training volunteers to support patients in their own homes. This was also a response to too few doctors, the challenges of covering rural areas, and the needs of those with cancer and HIV/AIDS. Volunteers provide practical, emotional, physical, and spiritual support to patients in their own homes involving members of the local community who speak the dominant local dialects. Evaluation of this programme reported the impact on patients and families, and how the CVWs acted as a 'bridge to the hospice' in identifying patients (Jack et al., 2011; Kiyange, 2014). Volunteers link patients with clinical teams when patients under their care experience serious symptoms including emergencies (Kiyange, 2014).

At the national level, community-based worker (CBW) systems can widen access to services and empower communities while also improving the outreach of services to those mostly underserved. Research indicates significant impact and sustainability potential through a community-based worker model (Khanya—African Institute for Community Driven Development, 2007). The study revealed that CBWs decreased the load on clinicians and extended their reach into communities. In Uganda, the Community Volunteer Programme augments the work of the hospice team by identifying patients living in rural communities not normally seen by the hospice team, or even knowing of the hospice or its work (Jack et al., 2011). A systematic review of end of life care volunteers indicated that volunteers take on a wide range of roles. These roles can be broadly classified into two categories: direct services for the patient; and supportive roles, including: administration, fundraising, drivers, gardeners, catering support, and general maintenance/housekeeping roles (Wilson et al., 2005). The role of volunteers in hospice and palliative care programmes is increasingly expanding from direct patient care to administrative, fundraising, and general support roles (Kiyange, 2014).

Other roles of volunteers include: household help for patients living alone; supporting child care givers through practical help in the homes; navigating health systems to facilitate patient access to services; and supporting patient triage and discharge plans at hospice and health facilities (Kiyange, 2014).

Motivations and success factors for volunteers in hospice and palliative care programmes

A number of studies have been carried out on volunteer motivation in the health sector in Africa. Topp et al., (2015) cite value-oriented functions; higher-order social aspirations such as 'helping society' or 'humanity' and economic and material support as motivations, while access to learning opportunities are also a key motivation for volunteering in hospice and palliative care. In Zambia, 11 per cent of the 758 caregivers surveyed indicated a desire to learn as their main motivation (Topp et al., 2015). Initial training of volunteers must be accompanied by refresher courses, follow-up, support, and mentorship as well as involvement in other hospice activities; in Uganda, these have been central to retaining volunteers. All volunteers need to have the knowledge and skills; also the supervision and mentorship to enable them to effectively execute their role (Kiyange, 2014). Volunteers are also motivated by having a staff volunteer co-ordinator as this shows that the organization has interest and values their work. This is usually a member of the paid staff who, as part of their role, coordinates activities of the volunteers. This staff volunteer works closely with an unpaid volunteer coordinator selected from among the volunteers themselves.

Recent Africa-wide research saw experts in hospice and palliative care iden-tify altruism, civic engagement, and personal gain (for a professional career) as having the most significant influence. Most volunteers received transpor-tation allowances or bicycles, some received small compensations. One in two experts noted that recruiting was easy and that cooperation with the commu-nity was often mentioned as helpful. Training mostly took place before the first assignment, with topics covering the palliative care concept, care, psychosocial support, and team work(Loth et al., 2015).

In South Africa, a monthly stipend has been found to enhance the sustain-ability of volunteer/CBWs' engagements. A stipend is a payment made to support living expenses of volunteers, unlike a salary paid to an employee. It is usually given to enable the volunteers meet their basic living expenses, as most of them have no source of income. Stipends are usually lower than what would be expected as a permanent salary for similar work. It is often distinct from a salary because it does not necessarily represent payment for work performed and cannot be measured in terms of a task. Where such a sti-pend is not given, the demands on CBWs can cause high attrition rates over the course of the programme. It is suggested that the feasibility of formalizing salary structures be explored (Khanya—African Institute for Community Driven Development, 2007). The issue of paying volunteers in hospice and pal-liative care programmes in Africa is a contentious one owing to the financial constraints of these programmes, which are mainly charity organizations. In some countries such as South Africa, volunteers have been integrated into the National Health Service through the integrated community-based home care model and monthly stipends are possible. Other countries remain far from implementing national policies and programmes that incorporate volunteers as paid members of health worker teams.

A study of volunteer AIDS caregivers' motivations in KwaZulu Natal in South Africa identified several motives with altruistic concerns for others and com-munity; employment or career benefits, and a desire by the unemployed to avoid idleness were frequently mentioned. The opportunity to learn caring skills or to put their own skills to good use for personal growth and to attract good things to themselves also figured. A few were heeding a religious call, hoping to gain community recognition, dealing with a devastating experience of AIDS in the family, or motivated for social reasons (Akintola, 2011). A study in Kenya identified some form of reward, be it financial or otherwise, in order to retain and maintain the engagement and motivation. This could be personal recognition, personal development, and working conditions (Takasugi and Lee, 2012). Facilitation of volunteers in African hospice and palliative care programmes is sometimes done by providing transport in form of bicycles, motorcycles, or other means to enable them reach the homes of patients (Kiyange, 2014).

Some individuals chose to volunteer as a result of caring for their loved ones using the knowledge and skills they had gained, while others are experienced patients who decide to contribute to the well-being of others with similar needs as themselves (Kiyange, 2014).

Research by Greenspan et al. (2013) identifies CHW motivation at the individual, family, community, and organizational levels. At the individual level, CHWs look to apply knowledge gained to their own problems and those of their families and communities. Families and communities bolster motivation by providing moral, financial, and material support, including service fees, supplies, money for transportation, and help with farm work and CHW tasks. Resistance to CHW work exhibited by families and community members is limited. The organizational level (the government and its development partners) motivates through stipends, potential employment, materials, training, and supervision, but inadequate remuneration and supplies discourage CHWs. Supervision can also be dis-incentivizing if perceived as a sign of poor performance. Tanzanian CHWs who work despite not receiving a salary derive motivation from familial support when other sources of motivation are insufficient. Training, work experience, networking, and the satisfaction of contributing to their community were cited as motivating factors for CBWs (Khanya—African Institute for Community Driven Development, 2007).

Comparing a study of volunteers in palliative care in India, where the basic motivation is a feeling of need to give back to the society to serve the sick and suffering, we find this very similar to findings from most studies in Africa. Other motivating factors identified were: team spirit, comfort shared, warm and respectful treatment by the team, satisfying nature of work, experience of cancer in the family, and aligned values and beliefs. Some intrinsic rewards mentioned by volunteers were joy of giving, personal growth, enriching experiences, and the meaningful nature of work (Muckaden and Pandya, 2016). The provision of required supplies such as protective gear to volunteers especially in situations of communicable diseases is also an important motivation (Kiyange, 2014).

Gaining social and political status at the community and national levels is becoming an important factor in decisions to offer voluntary services in hospice and palliative care. As volunteers become well known for providing a service, more of them are using this to establish and achieve political goals, such as being elected for a political position by the community. Providing the opportunity to volunteers to speak during public or community events is increasingly seen as a political motivation for them (Kiyange, 2014).

Challenges

The volunteering we describe here in hospice and palliative care and indeed in health care is an emerging field with a number of individual, institutional and system related challenges. For example, research in South Africa reported inadequate training, support, and supervision of community caregivers; random distribution of services leading to uneven coverage; poor integration of community home based care (CHBC) programmes with services offered by formal health facilities; and inadequate accountability by volunteers and their recruiting organizations (Caregivers Action Network, 2013). A recent Africa-wide study cites challenges related to funding and long-term motivation of volunteers (Loth et al., 2015)

Challenges affecting volunteers—financial and logistical?

Financial and logistical challenges exist in several countries. Topp et al. (2015) identifies work-related issues, client interests, caregiver interests and ambiguous interests as barriers to service delivery as well as failure to meet the expectations of volunteers. Failing to visit clients due to a lack of transport or to transport clients to health facilities were the most frequently cited barriers (73 per cent), followed by incomplete or unavailable homecare kits and supplies (35 per cent) and lack of weather gear, clothing and shoes (22 per cent) (Topp et al., 2015). Volunteers sometimes pay costs of telephone calls for people they are caring for out of their own pockets and should be reimbursed (Kiyange, 2014).

The lack of formal systems to manage volunteers work poses ethical challenges. Volunteers in Africa are generally poor and often HIV patients themselves. They often do not hold any binding contracts with their affiliate organizations, therefore do not have any form of work-related protection or financial and medical security (Kiyange, 2014).

Patients sometimes expect volunteers to be providers of food, as part of the package from their affiliate organizations/projects. When volunteers cannot do this it has often led to negative experiences, with volunteers feeling shame, ineffectiveness, and causing low morale (Topp et al., 2015).

Poverty is also a major challenge to hospice and palliative care volunteer services in Africa. Volunteers are often experiencing the same food insecurity as patients and in one study, the caregivers' own household food insecurity was explicitly cited as a barrier, an expectation not met, or both by almost one in ten respondents (Topp et al., 2015). The same study found 24 per cent of respondents citing own economic needs as a barrier, and 16 per cent identified economic needs as expectations not met by the project. Working without payment in the face of poverty is difficult for volunteers who have to return home with empty pockets despite some of them being patients themselves (Kiyange, 2014). Working with clients' poverty and sickness also caused CBWs stress (Khanya—African Institute for Community Driven Development, 2007). Another study found care organizations' poor understanding of volunteer motives a mismatch between organizational goals and volunteer motivations, and inadequate funding meant that volunteers' most pressing motives were not satisfied; in turn leading to discontentment, resentment, and attrition (Akintola, 2011).

Though volunteer work can help individuals obtain knowledge and skills ready for paid employment, research showed that retaining CBWs is difficult when the opportunity for paid employment arises, suggesting that a paid model might be a better practice (Khanya—African Institute for Community Driven Development, 2007).

National and organizational challenges

The absence of national and institutional policy frameworks, guidelines, and standards for the work of volunteers is a threat to the management of volunteers, especially in determining their workload. There is also a lack of monitoring of community care work, for example, where volunteers take on the work of employed staff. Personal risks such as assault and in some cases work overload among volunteers has been reported (Khanya—African Institute for Community Driven Development, 2007). Limitation of time and space due to the large volume of patients and maintaining continuous follow-up with the patients were reported in India, (Muckaden and Pandya, 2016), and these are also challenges in Africa. The lack of clarity of volunteer roles and conflicting expectations demotivates volunteers and sometimes role conflicts between volunteers and the staff of their affiliate organization arise (Kiyange, 2014). In South Africa, where new policy guidelines have been developed with a focus on state-employed community health workers, there are concerns this may lead to losing experienced community caregivers working in non-profit organizations (NPOs). This could also diminish the range of care and support roles that community caregivers based in NPOs give. Could home-based care no longer be provided if 'community health workers' became the only cadre of workers funded by the Department of Health? This would mean potentially losing day-to-day basic physical care and support for long-term bedridden and terminally ill clients within their home environment, long-term psychosocial support, assistance with securing livelihoods though accessing social grants or generating income, counselling, and regular drug adherence support (Caregivers Action Network, 2013).

The financial constraints at the institutional and national levels are also posing challenges for the formal integration of volunteers into health systems in Africa. Most hospice and palliative care organizations are charity based and rely heavily on external-donor funding which is dwindling. This is forcing organizations to scale down the very volunteer programmes that are critical in ensuring access to their services. In Uganda, a study of a Community Volunteer Programme reportedly showed this already happening (Jack et al., 2011). In Benin, Angola, Burundi, DRC, Congo Brazzaville, Cameroon, Chad, and Gabon, financial resources for health, and especially primary health care (PHC), have declined affecting community engagement (WHO, 2008). This means community health workers working without adequate resource support from either the communities they serve or from the health care system are further demotivated. The WHO has also noted that the supervision of personnel and their training/retraining in community health are inadequate and should be reinforced. Volunteers are expected to collect data and report on their activities, yet sometimes without adequate training and tools to enable them do this (Kiyange, 2014).

Work needs to be done to delineate boundaries between formal and informal community caregivers. Relationships between the formal health system and informal community caregiver programmes run by NPOs have not in the past been highly structured and often they depend on the individual efforts of staff in organizations and facilities. This limited degree of complementarity between formal and informal services needs to be addressed through policy guidelines (Caregivers Action Network, 2013).

There are also issues of volunteer distribution in countries. Some areas, especially the urban settings, are more served than the rural areas which affects the distribution of hospice and palliative care programmes in countries.

Some countries like Ethiopia have complex social and cultural context and this has financial implication on the recruitment and retaining of volunteers. Ethiopia has more than 80 ethnic groups, languages, and cultures. It is generally understood that essential services need to be delivered with community participation in ways acceptable and appropriate to this complex context (WHO, 2008).

Recommendations

Political and legislative

Governments need to be aware of the potential of volunteer initiatives and design their programmes accordingly. Community caregivers can effectively contribute to an expansion of HIV prevention, treatment, and primary care programmes, provided they receive adequate support, supervision, and training (Caregivers Action Network, 2013). This can be extended to the control and management of other disease conditions that require hospice and palliative care. Other issues that need to be addressed include: accredited training courses, how to make CBW systems more cost effective, and whether benefits to CBWs are adequate (Khanya—African Institute for Community Driven Development, 2007). African governments need to evaluate the cost saving on the involvement of volunteer workforce as well as understand key motivations for volunteer retention. Given the important roles volunteers offer, there is a need for governments and key partners to consider their inclusion in formal health and social service structures. This would necessitate the development of relevant policy frameworks, guidelines, and standards that should also address roles and motivational issues. India has been very successful in doing this and African countries can learn from them. Problems associated with lack of health personnel and their weak technical skills; insufficient financial resource allocation to the health sector, coupled with poor management of available resources can be addressed through the recognition, standardization, and monitoring of the status and work of community health care workers (WHO, 2008; Caregivers Action Network, 2013). The need to put in place a stock of reference documents and other management tools and introduce joint management options, cost-recovery methods, and incentive schemes for community workers is further recommended (WHO, 2008).

Reimbursement of volunteers

Findings from KwaZulu Natal in South Africa suggest rethinking current models of using non-stipended volunteers in informal AIDS care. Information about volunteer motivations could help organizations plan recruitment messages, recruit volunteers whose motives match organizational goals, and plan how to assist volunteers to satisfy these motives. This could reduce resentment and attrition among volunteers and improve programme sustainability (Akintola, 2011). It is further recommended that policy-makers and programme managers should consider the burden that a lack of remuneration imposes on the families of CHWs. In addition, CHWs' intrinsic desire to volunteer does not preclude a desire for external rewards. Rather, adequate and formal financial incentives and in-kind alternatives would allow already-motivated CHWs to increase their commitment to their work (Greenspan et al., 2013). The reimbursement of volunteers for costs incurred from their personal finances is specifically important, if no other financial incentives are considered (Kiyange, 2014).

Volunteering models and sustainability

Communities should be engaged at the early stages of conceptualization and design of volunteer programmes. The sustainability, reach, and output of volunteer programmes are enhanced by multi-stakeholder collaboration (Khanya—African Institute for Community Driven Development, 2007). Volunteer programmes in hospice and palliative care can derive important lessons from other non-health sectors in the country which involve volunteers in the delivery of their services such as in agriculture, forestry, water and sanitation, and natural resources.

It may also be cost effective for African governments to work with NGOs and evaluate existing models of volunteer service with the aim of consolidating or integrating them into one national programme or a harmonized and coordinated system that can serve both public and NGOs facilities (Kiyange, 2014). In 2010, the Government of South Africa launched new policy guidelines to revitalize its primary health care (PHC) approach with generalist community health workers employed by the state and deployed in outreach teams supervised by professional nurses and linked to formal health facilities in each electoral ward. Their main roles were defined as community profiling, risk identification, health promotion and education, and referral of clients to appropriate health services. Other important roles envisaged for the state-employed community health workers are to encourage people to test for HIV and TB and to support their uptake of and adherence to treatment.

Understanding the role and value of volunteers

Training to help hospice and palliative care organizations understand the role and value of volunteers is important for the effective management of a volunteers. Both the volunteer and the organizations will gain when volunteer roles are meaningful. Khanya recommends that facilitating and supporting organizations, the CBWs themselves, and the community must all receive training (Khanya—African Institute for Community Driven Development, 2007). Besides training, volunteers must be supported and supervised by professional staff. Policy makers and key partners must develop and fund home-based care models that take into account the stressors associated with AIDS care by reducing the work load, providing ongoing psychosocial support, and recruiting nurses to assist volunteers (Akintola, Hlengwa, and Dageid, 2013).

Volunteers also need access to very basic tools like reporting templates and referral forms (Kiyange, 2014).

Conclusion

Volunteers are an important resource in hospice and palliative care and need to be included in the development of such programmes by civil society organizations and governments. There is a wealth of evidence on volunteering in the health sector especially in HIV/AIDS care and support, which should inform volunteer programmes in hospice and palliative care. However, there is very limited research specific to volunteering in hospice and palliative care in Africa. The need for more comprehensive studies is evident. A key emerging issue is that of recognition and remuneration of volunteers by governments to ensure sustainability of such volunteer programmes in Africa. There is also a need for standard guidelines for hospice and palliative care volunteers that can be adapted or adopted by African countries to ensure quality services across the continent.

Formalizing the work of community volunteers in hospice and palliative care as well as wider health services is a critical issue for advocacy with African governments. South Africa and India can lend important lessons for the process.

References

African Palliative Care Association, (2011) *Standards for Providing Quality Palliative Care Across Africa*. Kampala, Uganda.

Akintola, O., Hlengwa, W.M., and **Dageid, W.** (2013) Perceived stress and burnout among volunteer caregivers working in AIDS care in South Africa. *J Adv Nurs* **69**(12): 2738–49.

Akintola, O., (2011) What motivates people to volunteer? The case of volunteer AIDS caregivers in faith-based organizations in KwaZulu-Natal, South Africa. *Health Policy Plan*. **26**(1): 53–62. doi: 10.1093/heapol/czq019. Epub 2010 May 28. Available from: https://www.ncbi.nlm.nih.gov/pubmed/20511348

Caregivers Action Network, 2013. *Community Caregivers: The backborne for accessible care and support multi-country research*. South Africa Report. Available from: https://www.cordaid.org/media/medialibrary/2013/09/SA_CAN_Report_26_July2013_3.pdf

Duwell, O.M., Knowlton, A.R., Nachega, J.B., Efron, A., Goliath, R., Morroni, C., Maartens, G.,and **Chaisson, R.E.** (2013) *Patient-Nominated, Community-Based HIV Treatment Supporters: Patient Perspectives, Feasibility, Challenges, and Factors for Success in HIV-Infected South African Adults. AIDS Patient Care STDS.* **27**(2): 96–102. doi: 10.1089/apc.2012.0348. Available from: https://www.ncbi.nlm.nih.gov/pmc/articles/PMC3565551/

Greenspan, J.A., McMahon, S.A., Chebet, J.J., Mpunga, M., Urassa, D.P., and **Winch, P.J.** (2013) *Sources of community health worker motivation: a qualitative study in Morogoro Region, Tanzania.* Hum Resour Health. **11**: 52. doi: 10.1186/1478-4491-11-52. Available from: https://www.ncbi.nlm.nih.gov/pubmed/24112292

George, A., Young, M., et al. (2012) Community health workers providing government community case management for child survival in Sub-Saharan Africa: who are they and what are they expected to do? *Am J Trop Med Hyg* **87**(Suppl 5): 85–91.

Jack, B.A., Kirton, J., Birakurataki, J., and Merriman, A., (2011) 'A bridge to the hospice': the impact of a Community Volunteer Programme in Uganda. *Palliat Med.* **25**(7): 706–15. doi: 10.1177/0269216310397566. Epub 2011 Mar 14. Available from: https://www.ncbi.nlm.nih.gov/pubmed/21402659

Khanya—African Institute for Community Driven Development, March 2007. *Final country report on Community-based Worker systems in South Africa.* Available from: https://assets.publishing.service.gov.uk/media/57a08bd7ed915d622c000f2b/8354_Final_SA_country_report_070723.pdf

Lehmann, U., and Sanders, D. (2007) *In: Evidence and Information for Policy.* Community health workers: What do we know about them? The state of the evidence on programmes, activities, costs and impact on health outcomes of using community health workers. Health DoHRf, editor. Geneva: World Health Organization.

Loth, C.C., Namisango, E., Powell, A.R., Pabst, K.H., Leng, M., Hamada, M., and Radbruch, L. (2015) *'From good hearted community members we get volunteers'—An exploratory study of palliative care volunteers across Africa.* (Unpublished.)

Muckaden, M.A., and Pandya, S.S., (2016) Motivation of volunteers to work in palliative care setting: A qualitative study. *Indian J Palliat Care* **22**(3): 348–53. doi: 10.4103/0973-1075.185083. Available from: https://www.ncbi.nlm.nih.gov/pubmed/27559267

Radbruch, L., Hesse, M., Pelttari, L., Scott. R., (2014) *The Full Range of Volunteering: Views on Palliative Care Volunteering from Seven Countries as Gathered in March 2014 in Bonn, Germany.* Bonn: Pallia MedVerlag.

Sepulveda, Cecilia, Habiyambare, Vincent, et al., (2003) Quality care at the end of life care in Africa. *BMJ.* **327**(7408): 209–13. Available from: https://www.ncbi.nlm.nih.gov/pmc/articles/PMC1126579/

Takasugi, T, Lee, A.C. (2012) Why do community health workers volunteer? A qualitative study in Kenya. *Public Health* **126**(10): 839–45. doi: 10.1016/j.puhe.2012.06.005. Epub 2012 Oct. Available from: https://www.ncbi.nlm.nih.gov/pubmed/23036777

Topp, S.M., Price, J.E., Nanyangwe-Moyo, T., Mulenga, D.M., Dennis, M.L., and Ngunga, M.M. (2015) Motivations for entering and remaining in volunteer service: findings from a mixed-method survey among HIV caregivers in Zambia. *Human Resources for Health..* doi: 10.1186/s12960-015-0062-y. Available from: https://www.ncbi.nlm.nih.gov/pubmed/26329324

Wilson, D.M., Justice, C., Thomas, R., Sheps, S., Macadam, M., and Brown, M. (2005) End-of-life care volunteers: a systematic review of the literature. *Health Serv Manage Res* **18**(4): 244–57. Available from: https://www.ncbi.nlm.nih.gov/pubmed/16259672

World Health Assembly (May, 2014) Sixty-Seventh World Health Assembly. *Strengthening of palliative care as a component of comprehensive care throughout the life course* [pdf]. Available from: <http://www.oeci.eu/Attachments%5CA67_R19-en.pdf>

World Health Organization (2008) *Summaries of Country Experiences on Primary Health Care Revitalization.* Report of the International Conference on Primary Health Care and Health Systems in Africa. Available from: http://www.afro.who.int/en/health-policy-and-service-delivery/

WHO, Fact sheet N°402, *Palliative Care*, (July 2015). Available from: http://www.who.int/mediacentre/factsheets/fs402/en/

World Health Organization (2001) World Health Report 2001. Mental health: new understanding, new hope. Geneva: WHO.

World Health Organization (2002) *National cancer control programmes: policies and managerial guidelines.* 2nd ed. Geneva: WHO.

World Health Organization (2016) *Planning and implementing palliative care services: a guide for programme managers.* Available from: http://apps.who.int/iris/bitstream/10665/250584/1/9789241565417-eng.pdf?ua=1

WHO Regional Office for Africa (2008) *Report on the Review of Primary Health Care in the African Region.* Available from: file:///C:/Users/fkiyange/Downloads/report_review_primary_health_care.pdf

Chapter 12

Volunteering in hospice and palliative care in India

Anil Kumar Paleri and Libby Sallnow

Volunteering and palliative care

With 1.32 billion people, India is the second most populated country in the world (UN Data, 2016). It is also said to be the land of contradictions (Sen, 2005). On the one hand, the country has successfully completed a mission to Mars, but on the other there are glaring inadequacies in the lives of millions, with 30 per cent of the country's populations earning less than 47 Indian Rupees (0.7 USD) per day (Planning Commission, India, 2014). India spends only 1 per cent of its GDP on health and more than 70 per cent of the heath needs are met by out-of-pocket expenses (Planning Commission, India, 2014). The efficiency of the health infrastructure varies across the 29 states and seven union territories and not all of them have palliative care as a priority. Three states (Kerala, Maharashtra, and Karnataka) have palliative care policies in place. Kerala has taken visionary steps to follow up the state policy declared in 2008 (Paleri, 2008) and has taken steps to integrate palliative care in to the health system. The government health institutions are central players in Kerala, along with non-governmental organizations (NGO). The state, with 3 per cent of the national population, is now estimated to have more than 90 per cent of the palliative care services in the country. This coverage is notwithstanding the fact that only 2 per cent of those estimated to require palliative care in the country have access to it (Kumar, 2013).

In India, palliative care programmes are often conceived and implemented outside health systems by NGOs, as a reaction to the inadequacies in the mainstream care for the dying and chronically ill, but this places the onus on the community for their development. Within the biomedical model of health care, which focuses mainly on the physical issues, the conventional response from most health institutions to people affected by incurable illnesses is, 'now we cannot do anything more for him/her, you can take him/her home'. This response can be considered to be a feeling of help-lessness which the community will also share as they watch their fellow beings suffer. So the question regarding what the community can do to im-prove experiences for those near the end of life is as relevant as questions regarding the health system's preparedness to address the issues of the chronically and incurably ill. Providing accessible and affordable palliative care to the more than six million people in India (Kumar, 2013; Murtagh et al., 2014) is a complex task and in areas where the community, through the volunteers, has shown a strong presence in palliative care, the coverage has improved tremendously.

Volunteering has long been considered an integral part of palliative care programmes, both in India and around the world, but there are varying extents to which volunteers participate in the process. In India numbers vary from state to state. Kerala is said to have trained between 150 to 200 thousand people and around 15,000 to 20,000 of these people are thought to be actively involved in the running of palliative care programmes in the state. In other states numbers vary and all together there will be a couple of thousand people actively volunteering in palliative care.

A case study: the Neighbourhood Network in Palliative Care

The Neighbourhood Network in Palliative Care (NNPC) in Kerala is an attempt to develop a sustainable, community owned service capable of offering comprehensive long-term care (LTC) and palliative care (PC) to those in need (Kumar, 2007). It was launched by four organizsations: the Pain and Palliative Care Society, Malappuram Initiatives in Palliative Care, Alpha Charitable Trust, and the Justice Sivaraman Nair Foundation in 2000, and represented a concerted effort to overcome the limitations of biomedical or professionally-led models of health care services. It is formed of a network of autonomous community initiatives, supported by trained palliative care professionals. The community and volunteers are empowered to take a leadership role in finding the solutions for the care of chronically ill and bed-ridden people in their own community.

The NNPC is inspired by the concept of primary health care as described in the 'Declaration of Alma Ata' by the World Health Organization (WHO) in 1978 (WHO, 1978), which describes primary health care as 'essential health care based on practical, scientifically sound and socially acceptable methods and technology made universally accessible to individuals and families in the community through their full participation and at a cost that the community and country can afford to maintain at every stage of their development in the spirit of self-reliance and self-determination.'

Traditional palliative care services, in India and overseas, are often run as services based in hospitals or as institutions. They can struggle to meet the needs of all those facing the end of life or requiring long-term care. The huge number of people needing such care, the complexity of social issues, the need for locally relevant solutions, and the requirement of care to be available 24 hours and seven days a week in people's homes, mean professionally delivered programmes often cannot provide the 'total care' people require (Twycross, 2007–8). The medical and nursing needs are just one part of a complex multi-faceted situation with social, emotional, spiritual, financial, and other issues affecting quality of life. Thus the needs of people requiring LTC and PC are identified as social issues with medical or nursing components, rather than the commonly held converse view (Kumar and Numpeli, 2005). To address these issues, the society is expected to take the lead and volunteers actively participate in organizing and running the programme. The network thus formed in the community will be available 24 hours a day as a 'safety net' to respond to the needs of the bedridden and chronically ill among them. It becomes less of a service and more a part of normal life.

The evolution of a typical palliative care programme based on the NNPC concept begins with a sensitization or awareness raising exercise in the community, in which as many interested people as possible are encouraged to participate. From these, a group composed of those who are ready and able to spare at least two hours a week for the cause are given a structured training programme. These 16 hours of interactive training include: discussion on the needs of people with chronic conditions; role of volunteers and the community in assessing and addressing needs; basics of communication; nursing issues; death and dying; organizing care in the community, and observation of home-care programmes (Kumar and Numpeli, 2005).

Trained volunteers then go on to form local groups to support people needing palliative care in their local area (Paleri and Numpeli, 2005). When fully established, community-based palliative care services are typically provided by both community health workers/volunteers and health-care professionals (WHO, 2016). Different programmes develop in different ways, depending on the resources, the skills the group possesses, and the pressing needs articulated by the community. Box 12.1 describes the different routes initiatives can take, emphasizing that there is not one prescribed route, but that all initiatives develop these key characteristics over time. For example, volunteers may start with a service providing only emotional and social support initially. Nursing and medical components may then be added later, with a home-care service when they are able to support the finances of paying staff.

Box 12.1 Action plan of the NNPC concept for developing community owned/based palliative care programmes

The Matrix of community-Based Palliative Care services consists of A. Medical Component, B. Nursing Component, C. Sensitised community volunteer, and, D. Trained community volunteer. The programme can start with any component and build the other components in due course (Kumar, 2015).

The protocol for developing community based palliative care programmes.

1. Sensitise the community; start social support programmes

2. Train volunteers and health care workers; start home care programme.

3. Get the services of a nurse

4. Get the services of a doctor

5. Set up out-patient/ in-patient care with trained nurse and doctor

6. Establish a system of regular review and evaluation

7. Repeat 1 and 2

Adapted with permission from World Health Organization (WHO). *Planning and implementing palliative care services: a guide for programme managers*, Copyright © WHO 2017. Available from: http://www.who.int/ncds/management/palliative-care/palliative_care_services/en/. Source: data from Kumar, S. Care Programs in Developing Countries and Role of Home Based Care in J. Thakur (ed) *Public Health Approaches to Noncommunicable Diseases*, Wolters Kluwer Health, Gurgaon, India, Copyright © 2015.

Understanding the role of volunteers within NNPC

Supporting a service versus owning a service

In the NNPC, the volunteers explicitly own the service. They are not working in a service run by others or a central office and they design and run the service adapted to their local community needs. This sense of owning rather than supporting can have a number of different impacts on how the work develops. One observation has been the extension of the remit of the service to areas traditionally considered outside of palliative care, such as support for patients undergoing dialysis, community psychiatry, and paraplegic patients. Volunteers describe how they see suffering and not diagnoses or diseases. The service reacts to the pressing needs of the community, and so providing a service that does not meet those needs does not make sense. This is one of the results of letting projects be driven by communities; they are more responsive to current needs but may challenge existing specialist definitions and boundaries. For this reason, the use of the term palliative care was augmented by long-term care, to cover the more inclusive nature of the work.

Follower versus leader

The change in profile of volunteers from followers to leaders also means that the tasks they take on also change. Many palliative care services are based in medical institutions and led by medical professionals, with only ancillary roles for volunteers. Organizations are able to survive without their support if needed. At the NNPC the volunteers become the pillars, rather than fillers, on whom the service is dependent. Except for the actual professional, medical, and nursing input, volunteers take up the lead roles in running the service.

Accountable to community versus accountable to funders

The funding for NNPC comes almost exclusively from micro-donations of a few rupees or less from people in the local community. This is one of the founding principles of the NNPC, in order to make the volunteers, doctors, and nurses accountable to those they are serving, rather than to external funders. This gives a freedom to act in response to the local needs rather than to externally imposed objectives. This accountability also acts as a quality control or safety measure, as communities are able to question services or the direction of the movement, if they do not feel it is representing or meeting the needs of the community.

Part time versus a part of life

The requirement of an NNPC volunteer is that they devote two hours per week to help those in need locally. Many volunteers work or have full-time jobs. They are teachers, bank employees, farmers, businessmen, and home-makers and volunteering in palliative care represents 'extra work' for them. But in another sense they are 'full time' volunteers who do not put a restriction on the hours in the week that they are available but are ready to help at any time, because they belong to the same community and live in the same area. In a sense they form a full-time 'safety net' in the community for patients and their families to fall back on if there is a crisis, and being a volunteer is a part of their life as a whole.

Younger versus older demographic

A striking feature of the volunteers in the NNPC is their relatively young age. This contrasts with the relatively older population of volunteers in programmes outside the NNPC. This difference in demographic composition has an impact on the type of activities that are undertaken by volunteers. Some clinics and home-care services are set up on university or college campuses and rallies and marches are often organized to raise awareness. Retired people make up an important component of the volunteer cohort but there is an interaction and vibrancy which comes from different parts of society coming together on a shared platform to address community challenges.

Engaged versus sensitized

A broad estimate is that NNPC network has trained around 150 to 200 thousand people up to 2016, but the number of volunteers who are actively involving in the programme is between 15000–20000 at any given point of time. Though it may look as if the attrition rate is very high, in reality the sensitized people form a part of wider network in the community. They help in spreading word about palliative care, directing people to services, support fund raising activities etc. As M. Sainudeen (personal communication, 3 August 2016), a volunteer put it, 'if the carer of an incurably ill person knows what palliative care is and how he/she can benefit from it, then there is a greater chance that the patient will get palliative care.' So even when they look passive, these sensitized volunteers will be contributing to the development of palliative care (Paleri and Numpeli, 2005). We feel that to keep more active volunteers, more and more people need to be trained. The active volunteers can be seen as the tip of an iceberg; the greater the number of sensitized volunteers in the community, the greater the number of active volunteers.

Direct patient care versus any role that will help

The scope of volunteering at the NNPC goes beyond the routine biomedical model of care that these patients usually receive. Apart from helping the patient and family accessing nursing and medical care, any other thing that could improve the quality of their lives can be taken on by these volunteers. This could include organizing financial support, buying medicines, supporting children's education, helping them access government support programmes, helping to access spiritual care, etc. Thus, anyone who can make a positive difference to the patients' and families' quality of life can contribute and palliative care is considered as 'everybody's business'.

Different models of initiating community participation at the NNPC

The foundation on which the NNPC concept is built is community participation. Once a community's participation is ensured it will further generate its own way of addressing the needs of the chronically ill among the community.

Since each community is different, assuming the Kerala model of community activation will happen everywhere may not be correct. Every community will need a catalyst element to activate the process of community participation.

Different models of community engagement other than the popular direct approach as used by the NNPC have been observed in India and the components of these differing models are outlinedin the next sections.

The NGO model

By far the most common way of ensuring community participation is to join hands with an NGO established in the area and with good community links. Examples are: The Sanjeevan Programme initiated by Institute of Palliative Medicine (IPM) in collaboration with the Sri Aurobindo Society at Pondicherry, and a programme initiated by in Cuddalore, Tamil Nadu in collaboration with Elder's Self Help Groups.

Local Government initiatives

The palliative care policy of Kerala rolled out in 2008 was heavily influenced by the existing community-based palliative care programmes (Paleri, 2008). This led to the integration of palliative care programmes into the government health system and now all the 1,076 Local Self Government Institutions (LSGI) in the state have primary palliative care programme. There was a perceived risk of losing the community ownership when palliative care is provided through the government system. With this in mind, the LSGI programmes were designed in such a way that community participation is ensured at the planning, execution, and monitoring levels of the programmes (Govt of Kerala, 2015). The elected members to the LSGI and Accredited Social Health Activists (ASHA), the trained female community health activists, also join the home-care programmes as volunteers. There is also active collaboration between the government programmes and existing palliative care programmes led by the volunteers.

Religious organizations

Compassion and care for the suffering is a core part of most religions and many religious organizations and institutions have adopted palliative care as an important activity. Though initiated by religious groups, their services are not limited to the people of the same religion and this has been an important avenue of growth for the NNPC (Sallnow and Chenganakkattil, 2005).

Political parties

The palliative care programmes have always enjoyed support from political parties in Kerala. This has led to the government taking an active stake in palliative care by rolling out a policy for the state and actively supporting it. Of late, some political parties have declared palliative care as a key interest. They are training their members in line with the NNPC concept and provide supportive care to bedridden people. They do not restrict the support to their own members and in many places collaborate with the existing programmes.

District administration

In West Bengal, a district administration, led by the District Collector (who was exposed to the NNPC concept during his tenure in Kerala) facilitated the process of sensitizing the community and setting up a multi-sectorial community initiative in Nadia district, led by volunteers, to provide palliative care.

Private hospital

In Manipur, the conflict-prone North-Eastern state, a private hospital has facilitated community participation. They have started by sensitizing the student community and the entire palliative care programme is now run by a network of more than 100 volunteers, mostly consisting of students.

Relevance beyond palliative care: the NNPC moving into other areas

The NNPC has developed into a significant social movement in Kerala and has inspired a range of further developments both locally and internationally. As NNPC volunteers recognize the impact their work can have, and develop this sense of agency, their attention will turn to other issues within society. This is an intended consequence of community development programmes—that the impact of the work is felt well beyond the immediate project. Two examples of this ripple effect are seen in Kerala. Palliative care services have collaborated with 'Mental Health Action Trust', an NGO for establishing a community care programme for people affected by psychiatric illnesses. Similarly programmes like the 'Footprints' Project at IPM have large-scale income-generating programmes for those who are bedbound and unable to work for a variety of reasons, to enable them to support themselves and their families (Institute of Palliative Medicine, 2010).

Compassionate presence

The Students in Palliative Care (SIPC) is a network of student volunteers aiming to bring the enthusiasm and energy of the student community in to palliative care and broader areas needing a compassionate presence. This highly motivated group become actively involved in the 'Compassionate Kozhikode', an initiative by the district administration to facilitate and provide a platform for 'sharing for betterment of people and places'. The strong sense of volunteerism developed by palliative care programmes in the district has been one of the motivators of the Compassionate Kozhikode initiative which has taken up tasks like: improving public places, supporting mental health centres, and children homes, feeding the hungry, and helping donors to find the right place (Compassionate Kozhikode, 2016).

'Samvedanam', is a recent initiative by Institute of Palliative Medicine and Compassionate Kozhikode, mainly targeting the younger population, aiming to give basic training in understanding the needs of the chronically ill and the dying. It supports the development of better communication skills so that they can be a compassionate presence to someone in need. This project, planning to train 2 per cent of the population in the district, aims at capacity building and doesn't seek active volunteering from the participants ('Samvedanam beckons youngsters to help sick', 2017).

Final reflections

The study of volunteerism in palliative care in India demonstrates multiple approaches, unsurprisingly, given the diversity of the country. There are large institutions that are not dependent on the community for financial support or for them to contribute significantly to the workforce. These palliative care services in big institutions like: All India Institute of Medical Sciences, New Delhi; Jawaharlal Institute of Postgraduate Medical Education, and Research, Pondicherry; and others, do not have a specific space for volunteers. They do try, however, to provide continuity of care through collaborating with the NGOs in the region. But there are other such large institutions as Kidwai Memorial Institute of Oncology, Bengaluru; and Tata Memorial Centre, Mumbai who invite volunteers to join them to provide care and support that the system is not otherwise able to give.

Then there are services run by NGOs who invite volunteers to join and support the programme by supporting those running it. In this scenario volunteers fulfill the tasks assigned to them by the administrators of the programme. It may be possible for a volunteer to join the decision-making group through a selection process approved by the organization but generally, in these programmes, they are not part of the decision-making processes. These institutions have varying degree of dependency on volunteers, but also will have a good professional system to support key activities like clinical services, administration, publicity, fund raising, etc. Most of the NGOs in the cities outside Kerala belong to this group.

There is an observed change from the perception of the West that older, more educated women generally volunteer (Goss KA, 1999). The NNPC has more young people as volunteers and there is almost equal gender participation. In the community owned/based programmes the volunteers and the beneficiaries are from a similar background but in big cities more volunteers are from middle and upper classes. The level of education of volunteers varies widely and the common motivation seems to be 'an inherent urge, a feeling of need to give back to the society' (Muckaden and Pandya, 2016).

Another interesting observation is on the influence of the caste system prevalent in India on volunteering. The palliative care programme in Pondicherry has observed that volunteers from lower caste are not welcomed in to upper-caste households during home care. In some places volunteers would restrict themselves to caring for the people from the same community or caste. Though the level of education and social stature of the volunteer can negate this to some extent, this phenomenon shows the challenges that wider community participation may shed light on, and the need for innovative approaches to address them.

Communities are not monolithic. Empowering communities comes with its share of confusion and anarchy. It was thought by the pioneers of the NNPC that palliative care would form a common platform, where those interested could meet whilst at the same time maintaining the pluralistic nature of the community. This did happen in many places but it was observed that close-knit groups such as religious and political organizations were also able to form such platforms for action. This may mean that one's personal beliefs and preferences are as important as shared feelings of compassion and responsibility in deciding which platform a volunteer would prefer to work from. We have further observed that this has created a subtle competition between services in the community. This may be good for the patient and family. Rather than polarizing the community and dividing the patient population, in a sensitized community, which can articulate its needs, the popularity and acceptance of a particular service will be decided upon by its quality. This may mean volunteers from different groups may have to redouble their efforts to meet the needs of community and will drive improvement.

Some organizations such as CanSupport, New Delhi and the organizations forming the NNPC, have clear volunteer enrollment and engagement plans. Most NGOs require volunteers to restrict themselves to palliative care activities but volunteers of some of the organzsations in the NNPC network have also taken up activities in related areas like supporting dialysis, prevention of non communicable diseases, and have also taken up social causes such as environmental issues. Purists may feel that this is diluting palliative care activities but the counter argument is that a socially active group has the freedom to respond to emerging social challenges in the community.

There are three main changes taking place in palliative care in India currently, since the modern hospice movement began three decades ago. The first one is the realization that chronic incurable illnesses are social issues with a clinical component (Kumar and Numpeli, 2005) and these social issues can be effectively handled by the community on their own, independent of the medical system (Stjernsward and Gómez-Batiste, 2008). This understanding widens the space for volunteers in palliative care to take a more active stake in the development and implementation of palliative care.

The second change is the greater ownership coming from government. With the National Programme for Palliative Care by the Government of India (2012) and palliative care policies announced by the Governments of Kerala (2008), Maharashtra (2013), and recently by Karnataka (2016) there is a greater onus on the elected leaderships and the governments themselves to act. Palliative care is no longer an NGO activity alone and 'Panchayati Raj' (Government of India, 1992), the decentralized governance system, potentially gives the common man greater say in developing locally relevant health-care programmes and participating in their implementation as evidenced by the LSGI-led palliative care initiatives in Kerala.

Thirdly, the changing way of understanding palliative care as a rights-based issue (Human Rights Watch, 2009) as against the commonly seen charity models is important. Instead of 'giving what you have', finding out 'what the patients need' and trying to fulfil those needs without disempowering people and compromising the dignity of patients and families through imposing what is 'thought to be' the right approach is now being appreciated.

All these areas invite greater participation from the community and will further promote the role of volunteers as providers and decision makers in palliative care programmes in the country.

Acknowledgements

We acknowledge the input from the following organizations in writing this chapter.

- All India Institute of Medical Sciences, Bhubaneswar, Odisha
- All India Institute of Medical Sciences, New Delhi
- Alpha Charitable Trust, Thrissur, Kerala
- Bangalore Baptist Hospital, Bengaluru, Karnataka
- CanSupport, New Delhi
- Delhi's National Initiative in Palliative Care, New Delhi
- Gangaprem Hospital, Rishikesh, Uttarakhand

- Government General Hospital, Ernakulam, Kerala
- Guwahati Pain and Palliative Care Society, Guwahati, Assam
- Initiative for Rehabilitation and Palliative Care, Kannur, Kerala
- Institute of Palliative Medicine, Kozhikode, Kerala
- Jawaharlal Institute of Medical Education and Research, Pondicherry
- Karunashraya, Bangalore Hospice Trust, Bengaluru, Karnataka
- KidwaiMemorail Institute of Oncology, Bengaluru, Karnataka
- Kozhikode Initiatives in Palliative Care, Kozhikode, Kerala
- Mental Health Action Trust, Kozhikode, Kerala
- National Health Mission-Arogyakeralam Palliative Care Project (from the 14 districts of Kerala)
- Pain Relief and Palliative Care Society, Hyderabad, Telangana
- Sanjeevan, Pondicherry
- Sanjeevani, Nadia, West Bengal
- Shija Hospital, Imphal, Manipur
- St John's Medical College, Bengaluru, Karnataka

References

Compassionate Kozhikode (2016) *Compassionate Kozhikode's Official Website* [online]. Available from: http://compassionatekozhikode.in/ [Accessed 30.01.2016.]

Goss, K. (1999) Volunteering and the Long Civic Generation. *Nonprofit and Voluntary Sector Quarterly* **28**(4): 378–415.

Government of India (1992). *The Constitution (Seventy Third Amendment) Act, 1992* [online]. Available from: http://www.nrcddp.org/file_upload/73rd%20and%2074th%20Constitution%20Amendment%20Act.pdf [Accessed 20.02.2017.]

Government of Kerala. (2015). GO (ORD) No.3217/2015/LSGI, dated 29 October. Thiruvananthapuram: Local Self Government Department, p. 50.

Human Rights Watch. (2009) *Unbearable Pain: India's Obligation to Ensure Palliative Care* [online]. Available from: https://www.hrw.org/sites/default/files/reports/health1009webwcover.pdf [Accessed 20.02.2017.]

Institute of Palliative Medicine (2010) *Report: Footprints, A pilot project for community based rehabilitation of the chronically ill and bed ridden*. Kozhikode: Institute of Palliative Medicine, p. 26.

Kumar S., and Numpeli M. (2005). Neighbourhood Network in Palliative Care. *Indian Journal of Palliative Care* **11**(1): 6–9.

Kumar S. (2007). Kerala, India: A Regional Community Based Palliative Care Model. *Journal of Pain and Symptom Management* **33**(5): 623–7.

Kumar, S. (2013) Models of delivering palliative and end-of-life care. *Support Palliat Care* **7**(2): 216–22.

Kumar, S. (2015) Care Programs in Developing Countries and Role of Home Based Care. In: J. Thakur, ed., *Public Health Approaches to Noncommunicable Diseases*, 1st ed. Gurgaon: Wolters Kluwer Health (India) Pvt. Ltd.

Muckaden M and **Pandya S.** (2016) Motivation of volunteers to work in palliative care setting: A qualitative study. *Indian Journal of Palliative Care* 22(3): 348–53.

Murtagh, F., Bausewein, C., Verne, J., Groeneveld, E., Kaloki, Y., and **Higginson, I.** (2014) How many people need palliative care? A study developing and comparing methods for population-based estimates. *Palliative Medicine* 28(1): 49–58.

Paleri, A. and **Numpeli, M.** (2005) The evolution of palliative care programmes in north Kerala. *Indian Journal of Palliative Care* 11(1) 15–18.

Paleri, A. (2008) Showing the way forward: Palliative care policy of the Government of Kerala.*Indian Journal of Palliative Care* 14(1): 51–4.

Planning Commission, Government of India (2014) *Health, Nutrition and Family Welfare.* [online] Available from: http:// http://planningcommission.gov.in/sectors/health. php?sectors=hea [Accessed 27.01.2017.]

Planning Commission, Government of India (2014) *Report of the expert group to review the methodology for measurement of poverty* [online]. New Delhi: p. 92. Available from: http://planningcommission.nic.in/reports/genrep/pov_rep0707.pdf [Accessed 28.01.2017.]

Sallnow, L. and **Chenganakkattil, S.** (2005) The role of religious, social and political groups in palliative care in Northern Kerala. *Indian Journal of Palliative Care.* 11(1): 10–14.

'Samvedanam beckons youngsters to help sick' (2017). Deccan Chronicle [online]. Available at: http://www.deccanchronicle.com/lifestyle/health-and-wellbeing/040217/kozhikode-samvedanam-beckons-youngsters-to-help-sick.html [Accessed 04.02.2017.]

Sen, A.. (2005) Contrary India. *The Economist*, [online] 18 Nov. Available from: http://www.economist.com/node/5133493 [Accessed 30 January 2017]

Stjernsward, J., Gómez-Batiste, X. (2008) Palliative Medicine—The Global perspective: Closing the know-do gap. In: Walsh, D., ed., *Palliative Medicine.* Philadelphia: Elsevier; pp. 2–8.

Twycross, R. (2007–8). Looking back and looking forward; Patient care: past, present, and future. *OMEGA* 56(1): 7–19.

UN Data. (2016). *Country profile- India* [online]. Available from: http://data.un.org/CountryProfile.aspx?crName=INDIA [Accessed 30.01.2017.]

World Health Organization (1978) *The Declaration of Alma Ata* [online]. Available from: http://www.who.int/publications/almaata_declaration_en.pdf?ua=1. [Accessed 15.01.2017.]

World Health Organization (2016) *Planning and implementing palliative care services: a guide for programme managers* [online]. Available from: http://www.who.int/ncds/management/palliative-care/palliative_care_services/en/ [Accessed 30.01.2017.]

Chapter 13

Volunteering and the challenges of change

Nigel Hartley

Introduction

We regularly hear about the key role volunteers have brought to the success of the modern hospice movement and of the importance Cicely Saunders attached to involving volunteers even before the first patients were admitted to St Christopher's Hospice in Sydenham in 1967 (Clark, 2002). Her rationale was visionary, for as well as filling a number of basic service roles; she saw two specific reasons why volunteer recruitment and deployment was fundamental to the hospice (Saunders, 1990). Firstly, she wanted to ensure that the volunteers reflected the patient and family population using the hospice believing this would offer security and familiarity to patients and families. The effect would be to make the hospice inpatient unit, although in many ways physically removed from the local community, still feel part of it. Secondly, she was keen that volunteers were also 'educators'; going back out into the local community and spreading the word to potentially change attitudes and perceptions towards the work that the hospice was doing, and, in doing so, also towards death, dying, and bereavement more generally. In many ways, 50 years later, Saunders' aims are still core reasons why hospices continue to involve volunteers as part of their service offering.

The UK is well known for volunteering and its attitudes towards it and as the Chapters 1 and 3 in this volume show, although the figures change if we take the 42 per cent figure for volunteering formally at least once during the previous year and 27 per cent for formally volunteering at least once a month (Institute of Volunteering Research 2014/5). This equates to around 21.6 m people and 13.8 m people respectively.

While it is difficult to accurately account for the number of people volunteering in order to support the work and mission of hospices in the United Kingdom (UK) (it is not unusual to find hospices do not have comprehensive records of volunteer numbers) Scott, 2015 (see Chapter 3) puts the figure at close to 160,000 volunteers.

Volunteers assist hospices in a variety of ways: for example, at Earl Mountbatten Hospice on the Isle of Wight, thousands of volunteers promote fundraising events in support of the organization. An 'Walk the Wight' event which has over 7,500 walkers attracts over 300 volunteers just for this event and for some this is the extent of their involvement. Many of our volunteers are in retail, the Earl Mountbatten hospice has ten community shops with hundreds of local volunteers involved as shop assistants, or collecting and sorting donations. Interestingly, the hospice also utilises the support of hundreds of prisoners from the island's prisons who offer support through upcycling furniture for our community shops, by sorting through clothes, or by making garden ornaments in their art and craft classes. In many respects, and uniquely, these prisoners are hospice volunteers though this also perhaps illustrates the fluidity with which the term volunteer can be used. Nevertheless, the wider the definition of volunteer the more we can agree that volunteers in hospices begin to truly represent a 'community of the unlike' all working towards a common cause (Saunders, 1990).

Hospices do, however, face new challenges as the introduction to this chapter implies and in order to consider these the Commission into the Future of Hospice Care (Hospice UK, 2013) was set up in 2011. One focus of the commission was the development and future of volunteering within hospices. A working paper (2012) reported on five recommendations:

1. Commitment to recruit a new wave of hospice volunteers
2. Establishing and evaluating training packages for local use
3. Hospice UK taking the lead on developing innovative and evaluated models of practice
4. National organizations testing more radical adaptations to current volunteering practice
5. More extensive research needed

The commission added a new energy to addressing the issues needing attention in the modern hospice movement, but it remains to be seen whether hospices on a local level can respond to the challenges and find creative and innovative ways of casting off the shackles of the past.

This chapter looks at the changes happening for volunteers supporting and working alongside clinical staff, patients, and families.

Volunteers and change

Most hospices offer a tried and tested model of care widely thought of as' the gold standard' of end of life care, that normally includes the provision of inpatient beds and a community multi-disciplinary team supporting patients and their families and friends in their home. Over the past thirty years, day care centres have become a common addition to in-hospice and home care. Hospices involve volunteers in all three of these areas—the hospice, the day centre, and the community, it is true to say though that involvement in the community has lagged because there is the unspoken benefit of keeping volunteers within sight of staff and volunteer managers and administrators within the hospice building. In essence, it provides a much simpler and potentially safer way of observing, supporting, and guiding the tasks that volunteers are expected to undertake. Therefore, on the one hand, the volunteer is valued and respected, and on the other most professional staff would rather keep them where they can see and control them.

Over the past 15 years or so, the traditional model of hospice care in the UK has increasingly come under scrutiny from a variety of sources (Randall and Downie, 2006). The majority of UK hospices remain as independent charities, and therefore could be viewed as being on the periphery of the health and social care system. Although there are many examples of partnership working with some hospices offering support to more mainstream health and social care organizations, the fact remains that, on the whole, hospices work mostly in isolation from the wider system, mainly due to funding models and their charitable status. There are many strengths and weaknesses to this particular model. From a positive perspective, and many believe this outweighs any negative impact, it is commonly accepted that there is a refreshing lack of bureaucracy which enables hospices to respond quickly to challenges with a speedy idea to action time which the main health and social care system might look upon with envy. However, a distinct vulnerability persists with remaining separate from the main health and social care system. The possibility of being overlooked as the system changes and develops around hospices is a common danger, as well as missing out on game-changing partnership opportunities and, above all, potential access to any new statutory funding. The pace of change within the health and social care sector continues to be relentless, and there is an increasing risk that if hospices do not continuously look outside of themselves, keeping their eye on the changing world around them, they could become obsolete and therefore irrelevant.

Some hospices are biting the bullet and innovating for the new world of health and social care (Hartley, 2013), but it is possible that the level and complexity of continuous change could threaten the very survival of many UK hospices.

A key challenge is that volunteers can hold much of the power within hospice culture. For example, at Earl Mountbatten Hospice, we have over 600 volunteers, together with just over 200 paid staff. Although at any one time we are supporting around 500 patients and families at home, most of our patient and family facing volunteers are involved within our hospice building, on our inpatient unit and within our day, self-help, and rehabilitation centre. This means at any time volunteers within our building can be the largest stakeholder group, albeit the size and membership of the volunteer group may change regularly. It is inevitable that with size comes power and influence. At a time of significant change the challenge persists of how we persuade and motivate a large stakeholder group, and one with the greatest perceived authority, to trust us and join us on a new and necessary journey.

Some personal examples

The following examples illustrate some of challenges I have encountered managing volunteers through organizational change in the five UK hospices I have worked in.

Example 1

At one hospice, we initiated a change programme within our hospice day centre, aiming to bring in more people who were interested in a 'drop-in' service than the old-style model of spending the day at the hospice. The drop-in service had a gym, a café and a number of support groups and attendees to the centre went up by 300 per cent. Despite preparing volunteers for this change, we found a group of long-term volunteers disliked what they saw as 'new' drop in centre users disrupting the routine of patients who had been, and were used to, spending all day at the hospice. We received a number of letters from unknown people within the local community voicing concern that volunteers were talking about leaving the organization because we had stopped really caring for our patients. They were threatening to go to the local press exposing us as having lost our way.

Example 2

At another hospice, a new training programme was set up for all existing and new patient and family facing volunteers to introduce and refresh their understanding of the hospice and what it did, as well as prepare them impending innovative changes in service delivery. A number of open meetings were held to explain the importance of the training programme to volunteers and a number of dates set to accommodate as many volunteers as possible. A group of long-term volunteers who had traditionally supported the inpatient unit categorically stated that they did not need training as they had been volunteering in their roles for long enough to know what they were doing. They refused to attend.

Example 3

During a time of change, a long-term volunteer made some unpleasant and derogatory remarks about senior staff in front of a group of patients, visitors, and other staff. A patient and their family complained to the hospice that the remarks were inappropriate. For the first time in its history the hospice had to use a disciplinary process similar to that which would be used with a paid staff member for the volunteer. During the process, it transpired that the volunteer had spoken inappropriately to a range of different people on other occasions. The volunteer, refusing to see their own behaviour as problematic, was asked to leave the organization. The volunteer went to the local press saying that she had been asked to leave because volunteers were being prohibited from speaking their mind and standing up for what is right.

There will be other examples from other hospices within the UK, but it is not usual that the complexities and challenges that are raised are articulated and understood more publicly. It seems there is an unprecedented fear from hospice chief executives, senior managers, and trustees about 'rocking the volunteer boat'. If not addressed and managed effectively and quickly, this fear could prevent hospices from transforming themselves into something more contemporary and relevant. There will be a number of ways of grasping the nettle to address the issues raised in the above examples, but the lesson is that to progress, as well as skill and experience, we will also require collective boldness, nerve, and confidence.

Experience shows that volunteers can be navigated better through change when there is a tangible reason for that change (Hartley, 2012). Examples may be refurbishment or rebuilding which provides an opportunity for things to be 'done differently', or a financial crisis where a lack of funding makes it clear that things cannot be delivered as before. Funding crises often mean brutal changes and different ways of behaving and practicing. At the time of writing the catalyst for change in the UK is the progressive failure of the wider health and social care system and its inability to do more for less whilst struggling with the imperative to innovate new models of care. This is echoed in growing demand and diminishing budgets in many hospices. How we achieve 'intimacy at scale' (Leadbeater and Garber, 2010), whilst offering solutions to local problems, as opposed to posing yet another problem to the wider system, will therefore be paramount for hospices.

Training, support, and partnerships

The Commission into the Future of Hospice Care (Hospice UK, 2013) was correct to highlight the need for establishing and evaluating new training packages, as well as promoting the value of volunteering and recruiting a new wave of helpers. Experience suggests this should be relatively straightforward. On the Isle of Wight we work with local schools and colleges to attract younger volunteers in their gap year(s) between school and choosing to go to university. While with us they gain experience in caring for patients and families prior to a potential career in health and social care. We continue to strive to recruit volunteers more locally to support people who are for example, frail and older, living with dementia, or dying within the locality that the volunteers live. We are fortunate on the Isle of Wight to still retain a sense of community and belonging within certain geographical areas. Developing this more community-oriented approach appears vital when all forecasts suggest many more people will become more isolated, lonely, and vulnerable and unable to remain within their own homes without simple, but skilled, day-to-day support. Projections suggest that, by 2035, three and a half million people in the UK will be aged over 85, one in three of them will die with dementia, and most with multiple chronic conditions (Dementia UK, 2016). The demography of the Isle of Wight means we will need to cope with this change sooner than the rest of the UK. The hospice, together with the whole health and social care system will need to develop services and support which will likely not be achievable without volunteers. A new Isle of Wight Volunteer Integration Group brings the hospice together with the local National Health Service and the national, but locally based charity, Age UK to explore how we might amalgamate and scale up some of our volunteer recruitment, training, and support structures to be more effective. However, the key to real partnership working will be how we articulate and agree what we are prepared to give away in order to achieve more together.

One blueprint could be the 2007 St Christopher's Hospice detailed training programme for patient and family volunteers (Hartley, 2012). Alongside this, the specific qualities needed by volunteers in order to support patients and their family members were articulated as:

◆ **Commitment to the hospice and its work and development**: attendance, punctuality and involvement in discussions and practice in training sessions

◆ **Self-awareness**: the ability to note your own behaviour, take responsibility for it and to change it where appropriate

◆ **Ability to communicate and listen**: the ability to express yourself so that others understand you and the ability to understand and respond appropriately to others

◆ **Ability to engage** with other people, individually and within the group

◆ **Being respectful** of others however different (or similar) they are to you

◆ **Willingness and flexibility** to undertake a range practical duties and activities

These qualities have also underpinned the development of our new training programme at Earl Mountbatten Hospice where formal training for volunteers has not been part of the agenda for a number of years. Many volunteers at Earl Mountbatten Hospice had felt unsupported by the lack of training opportunities, whilst others, albeit a small group, refused to believe that they need training at all. The new training programme is for all existing and new volunteers and all volunteers must attend. If some volunteers continue to insist that they do not need training, they will either be redeployed into non-patient and family-facing volunteer roles, or will need to leave the organization.

Example of six-week training programme

Key messages

We have worked hard to develop and articulate key messages to both staff and volunteers:

- Volunteers are a vital and integral part of the hospice team
- Without volunteers, we would not be able to offer the range and extent of services that we do
- Since the day it was founded, volunteers have made a dedicated and out-standing contribution to Earl Mountbatten Hospice
- We actively encourage the involvement of our volunteers within all areas of the hospice organization

The hospice has developed the new training programme for all volunteers who work in direct contact with patients and their families, or the general public. Examples of these include the John Cheverton Day Centre, Self-Help and Rehabilitation Centre the Inpatient Unit, the Patient Transport Service and the Home Visiting Service. A separate recruitment, selection and training process exists for any volunteers who wish to support our children, adult and family bereavement service.

Applications and interviews

Prospective volunteers complete an application form and a formal interview. The interview provides an opportunity for the applicant to reflect on their own motivation and understanding of what will be required of them. Successful applicants join the training programme prior to commencing any direct work, upon the receipt of references, an enhanced Disclosure and Barring Service (DBS) check, and an occupational health questionnaire. All existing patient, family, and public-facing volunteers are expected to undertake the new training programme which is part of the assessment process.

Training programme

The training programme is designed for volunteers who will provide direct support to clinical staff, patients, and their carers, and provides a comprehensive skill set for developing and sustaining the qualities, skills, confidence, and competence needed to be a hospice volunteer.

The training programme also varies teaching techniques so as to address different learning needs, for example: formal power point presentations, audio and visual examples of work with users, small and large group discussions, experiential exercises, role play, and 'hands-on' practice. Each session begins with a time for reflection using insights gained from the reflective diary process.

Evaluation

Feedback forms are completed at both mid and end points of the programme. Participants are also encouraged to share parts of their reflective diaries.

Assessment

Participants are assessed by the programme facilitator throughout the programme to ensure effective progression. Any concerns are raised directly with the participants and they are also expected to keep a personal reflective diary and encouraged to raise their own concerns at any time. Completion of the training programme does not necessarily guarantee that participants will go on to be a volunteer. All volunteers who go forward to practice have a formal 1:1 meeting after the first six months and then meetings at regular intervals.

Although there is a key person who facilitates the training programme, a range of other highly experienced hospice staff delivers specific sessions as detailed in Box 13.1.

Support and supervision

Volunteers are expected to volunteer for a period of one year following successful completion of the training programme. Although many stay longer than one year, it is understood that some may stop volunteering earlier than this for personal commitments. All volunteers are expected to attend a monthly support group session and a 1:1 meeting twice a year. All volunteers must also attend an annual update three-hour session for mandatory training purposes and undertake refresher sessions on current organizational vision and new projects. Other ongoing training is offered regularly during the year.

Box 13.1 Training programme sessions

Session 1: four hours
A. An induction to the hospice philosophy, and vision, and palliative care
Programme Facilitator
Member of hospice senior management team
Aims:

- To give an over view of the training programme
- To welcome and introduce the participants to each other
- Establishing the group's ground rules
- To give information about the history, vision, and current challenges of the hospice and palliative care
- To give information regarding ongoing assessment and expectations
- To give information about the role of volunteers supporting patients and carers

B. Impact of Serious illness: communication skills part 1
Programme facilitator
Aims:

- To explore the emotional and practical difficulties for patients and their families when managing serious illness
- To enable participants to put themselves in the position of a patient or carer and to acknowledge the different ways that people manage difficult situations
- To explore the ways users may be managing facing the end of their life and an uncertain future
- To develop listening and reflecting skills in order to enable and encourage users to communicate their needs

Session 2: four hours
A. Facing dying and death, support of patients' and their families as inpatients, outpatients, and in the community
Programme facilitator
Senior nursing staff
Aims:

- To acknowledge and explore fears of dying and death
- To explore the different ways people face the end of their life
- To provide an opportunity to ask questions about the physical process of dying and death and what happens to dead bodies

- To find out about how the hospice supports patients and their families as inpatients, outpatients, and in the community
- To provide information about how to support the nursing care of patients in different locations

B. Hospitality and customer care
Programme facilitator
Senior member of staff
Aims:

- To give information about the varying needs of users and visitors
- To give information about the resources available and how to recognize the needs of users and visitors and how and where to 'signpost' in order to access further support
- To explore assessment skills, develop awareness of individual needs, and practice ways of opening conversations with users/visitors
- To recognise the importance of hospitality and in providing high quality customer care

Session 3: four hours
A. Spiritual Care: communication skills part 2
Programme facilitator
Chaplaincy/spiritual care lead
Aims:

- To inform about the role of the spiritual care department and when it is appropriate to make a referral to them
- To give an overview of different types of funerals
- To enable volunteers to be aware of their own beliefs and to support users who have different beliefs to themselves
- To address concerns about managing silence when being with users
- To learn how to respond to users who are wanting to explore meaning
- To explore and acknowledge the differing needs of people who are dying
- To develop communication skills which help users to feel understood and accepted whatever their feelings and thoughts on reaching the end of their life

B. How to help people access information and give feedback
Programme facilitator
Senior member of staff

(continued)

Box 13.1 Continued

Aims:

- To develop skills in supporting users to access useful and supportive information via the computers/ internet and leaflets/ booklets
- To inform about the range of information that users could access: e.g. health, benefits, funerals, wills, supporting carers
- To develop skills in responding and encouraging user feedback and be informed about how the hospice uses feedback
- To complete the mid-point evaluation

Session 4: four hours
A. Supporting nurses: care of patients
Programme facilitator
Member of the nursing team
Aims:

- To learn how to best support the nursing staff
- To learn about the safest way to feed patients
- To practice feeding and to experience being fed

B. Grief and Bereavement: children and young people
Programme facilitator
Aims:

- To inform about the needs of bereaved people and how to support them
- To learn about how the hospice supports bereaved people
- To learn about children and young people's needs and how to respond to them and provide support
- To inform about the hospice and how it supports dying children and young people as well as bereaved children and young people

Session 5: four hours
Supporting people at home
Programme facilitator
Senior member of staff
Aims:

- To give information about how the home visiting service works and how users can access
- To gain an understanding of this role

- ◆ To develop self –awareness and skills to support patients at home
- ◆ To develop self-awareness and skills to support at home

Session 6: four hours

A. *Communication skills part 3*

Programme facilitator

Member of personnel, staff

Aims:

- ◆ To inform the participants of relevant policies, hospice practice, and management structure
- ◆ To develop skills in assessing how to the differing needs of patients and their families
- ◆ To practice a range of communication techniques which meet users' needs

B. *Looking after yourself: accessing support and supervision*

Programme facilitator

Senior member of staff

Aims:

- ◆ To provide information about the support, supervision, and future training available
- ◆ To congratulate and welcome the volunteer to their new role
- ◆ To provide information about the systems and structures of volunteer rotas and shifts
- ◆ To give an opportunity to explore hopes and fears about the new role

Short-term placements

Short-term placements are also available. An example of this is someone who wishes to go on to study medicine or other health and social care related professions and might benefit from a few days volunteering at the hospice. As with other volunteers, an application form and face-to-face interview are required, if successful, they then have a brief induction session by the manager of the department in which they volunteer and are attached to an experienced volunteer for the duration of their short-term placement.

A group hospice introduction programme is also available to schools, colleges, and other organizations. Groups have the opportunity to experience different areas of the hospice organization, including the John Cheverton Day Centre, Self-Help and Rehabilitation Centre, fundraising, shops, etc.

New developments

In the near future, we plan to include:

1. **Discharge support from the local hospital or the hospice**—Many patients and families find discharge from inpatient services extremely problematic. A volunteer will provide help with 're-socialization'

2. **Care Home Support** –We are also committed to improving the quality of end of life care in Care Homes. We aim to act as a 'hub' for providing community support volunteers, alongside staff who are already offering some support and education, into a number of care homes across the island

Content analysis of recent evaluation

Content analysis of evaluations undertaken during the first three volunteer training programmes at Earl Mountbatten Hospice highlighted four main themes:

1. Belonging and feeling included
2. Expertise of staff
3. Understanding of change
4. Motivation and determination

Some feedback examples include:

1. Belonging and feeling included

   • 'It feels such a relief to know and understand where the organization is going and why…I feel that I really belong again after being out in the wilderness…'.

2. Expertise of staff

   • 'The staff who have taught us are all on board with the changes and new direction…if it's good enough for them it's good enough for me'.

3. Understanding of change

   • 'I am getting old myself, and I am reassured that even if I die from something else other than cancer, the hospice will endeavour to be there'.

4. Motivation and determination

   • 'I am a new volunteer, and it has been interesting to hear the experiences of those volunteers who have been around for a while …I have learned that I can make a difference and support patients and families wherever they happen to be…'.

As with all feedback, there was of course some constructive criticism which we will address as the future evolves.

Conclusion

This chapter began by highlighting Cicely Saunders' approach of involving volunteers from within the local community, reflecting the patient population, and acting as ambassadors through public education. If this remains the case today, then the views of volunteers must surely partly reflect the views of those members of the local community who are relying on our support as they come to die and those members of the local community who support us through donations and fundraising efforts. It will also be inevitable that the messages volunteers take back to their communities will reflect their own experiences of the hospice.

The challenges of managing volunteers through change are many and varied and wider even than those mentioned throughout this chapter. Any new approach towards hospice and palliative care volunteering has to be driven by the necessity for a new and transparent set of agreements between ourselves, existing and potential new volunteers, together with members of our local community. A clear set of jointly agreed and articulated expectations, and an insistence on continuing to develop thorough and well organized recruitment, training and support structures will also be paramount.

The process of change for hospices, where they will need to reform and remain relevant through continuing to revolutionize care for all dying people and their families, whoever they are, whatever their circumstances, and wherever they happen to be, will certainly persist for the foreseeable future. The involvement of volunteers in this process will be crucial to success. The measure of this success might very well yet depend on our ability to innovatively and boldly renegotiate terms and expectations with one of our largest stakeholders, our volunteers.

References

Clark, D. (2002) *Cicely Saunders Founder of the Modern Hospice Movement Selected Letters (1959–1999)*. Oxford: Oxford University Press.

Dementia UK https://www.dementiauk.org/understanding-dementia/ [Accessed 06.2016.]

Hartley, N. (2013) *End of Life Care: A Guide for Artists, Therapists and Arts Therapists*. London: Jessica Kingsley Publications.

Hartley, N. (2012) Volunteering at Saint-Christopher's Hospice, London: Current trends and future challenges. In: *Medicene Palliative, Soins de support—Accompagnement—Ethique*. Volume 11. Elsevier Masson: France, (pp. 252–61).

Hospice UK (2012) *Volunteers Vital to the Future of Hospice Care A Working Paper*. London: Help the Hospices.

Hospice UK (2013) *Commission into the Future of Hospice Care*. London: Help the Hospices.

Institute of Volunteering Research. Available from: http://www.ivr.org.uk/ivr-volunteering-stats. [Accessed 06.2016.]

Leadbetter, C. and Garber, J (2010) *Dying for Change.* , London: Demos.

Randall, F. and Downie, R.S, (2006) *The Philosophy of Palliative Care: Critique and Reconstruction.*, Oxford: Oxford University Press.

Saunders, C. (1990) Hospice and Palliative Care An Interdisciplinary Approach. London: Edward Arnold.

Scott, R. (2015) We cannot do it without you—the impact of volunteers in UK Hospices. *European Journal of Palliative Care* **22**(2): 80–3.

Chapter 14

Volunteering and community

Libby Sallnow and Heather Richardson

Introduction

Volunteering and 'community' are two concepts that are often closely aligned in hospice care. The number of volunteers working on behalf of hospices is often cited as in excess of 160,000 (Scott, 2015), their motivation driven, at least in part, by being part of the local community served by the hospice. These individuals understand that a set of reciprocal relationships exist between those who need expert help at the end of life or in bereavement, organizations skilled and resourced to respond, and the community on whom the hospice draws to support its response. There is no greater evidence of this relationship than the presence of over 220 hospices in the UK that sit within the voluntary sector. As discussed in Chapter 3, many of these hospices were set up by individuals and groups present within a local community who identified a gap in end of life care services and set about galvanizing support and raising funds to create a new resource for themselves, their families, friends, and neighbours. They drove efforts to build new facilities and establish professional teams, as a means of achieving their vision for high quality, local, end of life care. Volunteers have perpetuated such efforts in subsequent years by playing key roles in funding and delivering hospice care in their area, alongside a paid workforce.

Health, community, and volunteering

In recent years, the role communities can play in health has received increasing attention. There is strong evidence within the literature that community participatory approaches, such as health promotion, social networks, community development, and engagement can have a positive impact on wellbeing, survival, and a range of other health outcomes (South, 2014; O'Mara Eves et al., 2013). As a result, these approaches have increasing traction within health and social care (National Institute for Health and Care Excellence, 2014). End of life care has been no exception. Health-promoting palliative care and compassionate communities, two approaches that encompass community development principles, enjoy growing attention within the sector (Kellehear 2005; Karapliagkou and Kellehear, 2014). Numerous examples of how they work in practice now exist internationally (Sallnow et al., 2012; Wegleitner et al., 2015).

Community and volunteering—through the eyes of volunteers

This chapter focuses on a group of volunteers that support individuals who are dying or bereaved and through their efforts attempt to change the wider community in which they live. We will explore their experience of volunteering, their motivations for this work and how this fits with their views and beliefs about community. We will also identify some of the impacts identified as a result of this work. It draws on doctoral research undertaken in East London, aimed at evaluating a volunteer-led initiative to provide support to individuals who have serious or life-threatening illness. It focuses specifically on the positive impact and facilitators for this work. The organizational challenges and barriers to this work are considered elsewhere (Sallnow et al., 2017). The content and analysis of interviews with volunteers forms the basis of the snapshots we offer of the volunteers and the themes emerging regarding the impact of this work and its facilitators and barriers. Their detail has been negotiated with them. The detail of this research and its broader findings relating to stakeholders beyond volunteers is described elsewhere (Sallnow et al., 2017).

We begin by describing this initiative and its aims; then we introduce three volunteers who are involved in its work and comment on their perspectives and those of other volunteers who have also been interviewed as part of the research. Finally, we consider the emerging themes in relation to the notion of 'community' and offer some reflections on the fit or otherwise.

Introduction to the service—Compassionate Neighbours

The Compassionate Neighbours project was set up by St Joseph's Hospice in 2013 as part of its care offered to the people of Newham, Hackney, and Tower Hamlets. It was a direct response to the requests of local people, and particularly members of particular black and minority ethnic groups (BAME) groups who, on consultation with the hospice, had identified gaps in provision available to their families, communities, and neighbours when they were seriously ill or dying. The programme of engagement and consultation, described elsewhere (for example Richardson, 2012) was informed by a community development approach offered by a partnership organization called Social Action for Health. It highlighted opportunities for improved public education and understanding about the processes of death, dying, and loss, different models of care, and amended policy and practice following death, such as certification and requirements for post-mortem examination. In relation to models of care, requests were made for support that addressed the social, as well as the clinical needs arising from a terminal diagnosis. Such a suggestion made by someone from the local Bengali community, cited in Richardson (2012) describes the detail of such support:

> We need volunteers that can, perhaps, go with the home care team into people's homes. These volunteers don't have to talk about the illness just provide support to patients and families in their own language because sometimes its difficult for patients or families to talk to either other family members or service providers about certain issues. But it's easier to talk to someone from the same cultural and religious background who speaks the same language. That would have really helped when my father-in-law was dying at home.

The compassionate neighbours programme seeks to address these needs. Carefully trained and supported volunteers—known as compassionate neighbours, drawn from local communities enroll in a training programme run over a series of weeks at the hospice. This training focuses primarily on personal reflection and growth, confidence building, awareness of the principles of community development and compassionate communities, and crucially, the development of a strong peer support network. Policies such as safeguarding and confidentiality are taught: but the training aims to develop flexible, creative, competent, and self-aware people able to act as neighbours to others in the community. There is not a binding role description, but rather the compassionate neighbours are taught to determine what the person might need and tailor any offer of support around this. The choice of the term 'neighbour' was intentional; it is a role familiar to people and it means volunteers do not run the risk of becoming 'professionalized' into health or social care roles.

Compassionate neighbours complete a Disclosure and Barring Service (criminal records) check and are then matched up with individuals who are seriously ill, or their carers—known as community members. The terminology was again important here. The compassionate neighbours discussed the different terms used to describe those usually using a service such as service users, beneficiaries, patients, or clients and felt none reflected their place within this project. Eventually the term 'community member' was agreed upon. This was felt to reflect the fact that these were people just like the volunteers, often self-referred into the service or referred in by other members of the community and often outside any interaction with health and social care professionals. The use of other terms was felt to imply a hierarchy of need and power between two people coming who were in fact coming together to enjoy mutual support.

The match between compassionate neighbour and community member takes into account ethnicity and language, interests, geography, and availability and has no time limit. Further to this, compassionate neighbours have a role in building bridges between local people and communities with the hospice, training and supporting other neighbours, and looking more widely at how the local community could be supported to become a more compassionate place to live and die. The relationships established are focused on extending mutual support and kindness. Some of the help on offer may be practical in nature as well as emotional. This is negotiated and shaped within the relationship, assisted and monitored through regular practice-development meetings of the compassionate neighbours who offer advice and comment to their peers. These monthly meetings, to which all compassionate neighbours are expected to attend, focus on the detail of the narratives or stories offered by the neighbours regarding the relationships that they are developing, their triumphs and challenges and what opportunities this presents for self growth and learning, alongside the support provided.

In the first two years of the life of the project, over 180 people have been recruited and trained as compassionate neighbours. They have been matched with 70 community members and together they represent the beginnings of a growing and thriving social movement that aims to change how people live and die in the East End of London. Since the inception of this service, St Joseph's has been successful in securing additional funds to support the work, has recruited two full time members of staff to lead the project, both with community development backgrounds, and has participated in a number of research and evaluation projects. At the time of writing it is seen as a major part of the life of the hospice and as a crucial part of its work to continue to improve end of life care for the people of East London.

Introduction to some of the compassionate neighbours

Pat

Pat, an older AfroCaribbean woman, first heard about compassionate neighbours when someone from the hospice came to a lunch club to talk about how people deal with death and dying and what role communities can play. Pat remembers thinking that she 'knew she had compassion, but as to becoming a compassionate neighbour, that was a different thing for me…'. She had first-hand experience of being a carer for a family member and was aware of the limited support other family members could offer. She did not want to burden already busy children so carried on alone and became progressively more isolated. Being introduced to the concepts of compassionate neighbours and completing the training afforded her a new perspective on community and gave her the confidence to seek out further volunteering opportunities. She now sees herself as a connected member of the community and is an integral member of many other projects supporting people with mental health issues and women using maternity services, all following on from this first opportunity.

She has supported two community members and sees her role as providing something that neither professional services nor family can provide. The unique position of not trying to change or influence the situation of the community member or to deliver a service means she is free to meet the person where they are and support them as they are. As she is a peer of the community members, she feels there is reciprocity in the support—it could easily be her sitting in their chair—and this guides her sensitive and individualized care.

One of the unexpected outcomes of the training for Pat was the dispelling of the myths she had held about the hospice. The project has led her to be a 'foot soldier of the hospice'—going out into the community to share the positive message of the support and care that is available for people at the hospice and challenging views held, particularly in communities not accessing the service. Pat feels that the support of a hospice is important for compassionate communities projects but also that hospices are incomplete without the support of communities in this practical and engaged way.

Kathy—who tells her own story

I first got to know the hospice when they offered to host our Older Lesbian Group meetings we were holding, which were looking at how we could support each other as we became older. I felt welcomed by the hospice and wanted to do something in return. When the opportunity to enrol in compassionate neighbour training was announced, I thought that this would be a good way of giving something back. I am deeply committed to the principles of engagement, access and equity that underpin the work and it was this is what made the project seem particularly attractive. When I started training I realised that being part of this was a real opportunity for me to work within a feminist perspective around social change and this was really exciting.

I now visit an elderly isolated man and have developed a close relationship through sharing conversation, being a regular part of his life and developing trust. I support him with a range of issues he is living with. As part of the wider perspectives of compassionate communities work, I have begun to look at how we can find broader solutions to social isolation in this local area and I have begun to work with others to begin to change the experience of people locally.

The unique aspect of compassionate neighbours for me is the empowering nature of the work. I feel it is different to other volunteer roles I have done, as the training works to develop our autonomy and we are able to work flexibly with our community members to do what is needed for them, rather than being bound by a specific job description or restrictive risk management. This requires experienced and flexible management but the results are real change in the lives of the community members we are matched with and significant changes for me as a person. I feel a sense of hope and purpose from being part of this. Hope that we can change the experiences for the community members we see and as part of a social movement change the community we live in. The sense of purpose this gives me in some ways replaces the sense of purpose I had when I was working, and this is important in making my life full and meaningful.

Kito

Kito, a 47 year old man originally from Laos, was a successful chef when his son was diagnosed with autism and he became a full-time carer for him. He describes how his life gradually contracted until he had very limited social contact beyond appointments and assessments and he had lost hope about anything changing in the future. He heard about compassionate neighbour's training at a carers' week event and was unsure about applying. In the first few sessions he was very quiet and shy but describes an 'explosion' a few weeks in where the work began to resonate with him and he discovered a reason to get up in the morning. He made a strong network of friends in the training and this led to his confidence improving. He describes how his phone was once silent but now is busy with calls and texts from friends and social plans.

Kito was matched with a socially isolated older man who had not left his flat in many years and saw no one aside from his carers. He and Kito quickly found a series of shared interests and talked animatedly through their first meetings, despite both being nervous about being matched up. Kito has been helping his community member develop his confidence in going outside; they recently went to get a haircut together and often see each other a few times a week. Kito is animated when he talks about his relationship with his community member and the strength of the relationship that has developed.

He feels he has gained a friend and found new meaning, skills and happiness through this work. 'I have so much confidence now. I have learned to listen to people and let them do the talking. I really think that the compassionate neighbours training has helped with my son too; he has come on really well and I have learnt that patience really pays off. With my new found confidence I am planning to do some cookery teaching. Sushi is my speciality and I already have some classes lined up. Both [community member] and my son are definitely happier than before. I put that down to my compassionate neighbours training. It has really changed me for the better'.

The impact of this work on volunteers

Through their stories and those of other compassionate neighbours, we are able to identify some ways in which this work has impacted their lives.

The first is *change in attitudes*. Pat described how her experiences had made her consider on her own mortality and reflect on her wishes should she become unwell. They also challenged her long-held views about the hospice, previously believing it was a 'dead-end place' whose name was to be said in a whisper, to believing this was a resource the whole community should know about, that it is 'part of the living community' and she has a role in spreading this message. Compassionate neighbours spoke about how the experience of being part of this diverse community, focused on the highly personal processes of death, dying, and loss had enabled them to respect and enjoy difference between individuals and groups. This notion of tolerance and openness was again described by Pat, 'community now for me is something different ... I'm not afraid of sitting among the people'.

The second theme is about *personal wellbeing*. Numerous stories were shared by compassionate neighbours about how joining the project had dramatically changed their lives. Kito describes being relatively isolated before joining the project and of the project 'revolutionizing' his life. The peer network that is created in the training and is developed further in monthly practice development meetings created a sense of belonging, of purpose, and of value. In this way, the training serves as an intervention and an end in itself, where members of the community learn from, and connect with each other. Many of the compassionate neighbours, like Kito, described 'feeling happy' at having the project in their lives. Kathy found that even with a full and busy life, she was surprised at how the project had enriched it. Compassionate neighbours described how this work has served as a springboard for further opportunities—employment or further volunteering —due to the confidence and broadened perspective gained.

The third theme relates to the creation of *new relationships*. These exist between the compassionate neighbours and their community members; small peer groups of neighbours, and the community of compassionate neighbours as a whole. As a result the neighbours enjoy new connections with individuals, institutions, and different groups of people. These relationships and the trust, intimacy, and respect that they include represent the notion of social capital as described in the literature (Szreter and Woolcock, 2004). Through this we see evidence of bridging social capital (which describes the relationships between heterogenous groups within communities) and linking social capital (those relationships between communities and their institutions) (Baum and Ziersch, 2003).

Facilitating volunteer involvement in community developments

Most important is the opportunity for compassionate neighbours to *learn as a community*. Compassionate neighbours were able to describe how they were the 'first partakers in what we were offering'. They were not required to bracket off what they were experiencing in their personal lives during training, but encouraged to share it and to build the capacity of the network to support them through it. At the end of each training session, the whole group ate together and this was part of the training costs. At the start, some compassionate neighbours did not understand this and thought it was a waste of money, but it was a key requirement by Social Action for Health. As the course progressed and relationships deepened through sharing meals together, the importance of valuing people through sharing food together was recognized and it is a key part of meetings.

The training and indeed the whole programme must be driven by a *unifying vision and purpose* that captures participants' imagination and motivates them to take part. This is broad in nature, enabling people to find a place for their particular driver to be involved. The wider purpose of initiating a social movement is important to many, lending a broader significance to the work, beyond one-to-one visiting, and leading to feelings of empowerment and agency—feeling that real change is taking place due to their actions.

Once trained, compassionate neighbours are free to adopt *a role that is responsive* to the community member's wishes and needs and reflects the compassionate neighbour's strengths. Compassionate neighbours felt that their role, having no overt agenda other than to accompany the community member on their journey and be there for them, allowed them to develop a close and trusting relationship which sat separately from paid carers and professionals, and from family members, and importantly allowed them to meet needs not met by these other groups.

As a result, their work is not based on dependence and passivity on the part of the community members and specifically is not a service. The concept of *mutuality and reciprocity* emerged again and again, where compassionate neighbours were able to articulate that they were getting as much out of the match as the community member, that they were peers supporting each other in reciprocal ways and that life could easily change, such that they would be 'on the other side of the door'. This empathy and sense of a real relationship being formed appeared fundamental to the success of the project.

The link with the hospice was important. It lent a *legitimization to the caring role* they were taking on and offered them a related sense of authority. Many people had wanted to reach out to neighbours nearby but were worried about just knocking on their door. By working with the hospice, the compassionate neighbours felt more confident to make this offer. This helps to illustrate the role a hospice or other organization plays in developing such an initiative.

Finally, leadership that draws on *community development principles* is crucial. The leader must be able to articulate the vision for the work and inspire and motivate those who may have never considered a volunteering role to date. They must be able to manage and hold risk and uncertainty and create a space in which people can discover their own potential and the opportunities open to them to make a difference to others and their own lives. This work is complex, but it must remain flexible and organic in approach, allowing real relationships to develop between individuals. Attempts to prescribe processes and outcomes limit the work and can restrict it to a service offering companionship.

Reflecting on these experiences and the notions of community and volunteering

The experience of volunteers

The stories of these three individuals who work as compassionate neighbours highlight the broad nature of their experience as volunteers. Along with other compassionate neighbours interviewed by Sallnow, they describe an experience of social and personal transformation—achieved through new relationships, and a different view of self. They, and other compassionate neighbours, make new friends; they recognize the contribution that they can make to the lives of others and enjoy a new found sense of agency and empowerment. Their relationships are those of mutual support—including the relationships that they have with their community member and other compassionate neighbours. The relationship they build with the hospice is important, offering a sense of belonging and a legitimization of their role.

At the heart of their learning and highly positive experience of being part of this initiative is the training that they participate in. The training that compassionate neighbours received places their growth and personal development at centre stage and importantly as an end in itself. It offers participants the opportunity to be seen as community partners, recognizes that they have expertise in areas that professionals do not, and places priority increasing the capacity and resilience of communities in the face of death, dying, and loss. This would appear to be in contrast with more traditional hospice volunteering role, which is often focused on helping the hospice achieve its aims. According to the literature, these include: extending the range of services available to patients and carers; supporting staff to carry out their duties; and undertaking specific roles within the hospice, such as gardening, or reception work, or fundraising, and raising awareness of the work of the hospice locally (Burbeck et al., 2014). Although volunteers are highly valued members of the hospice workforce and have access to training, their development is not the primary goal of the relationship. Whilst this chapter has focused on compassionate neighbours as volunteers, and indeed some compassionate neighbours describe themselves as such, the authors are left reflecting on the degree to which their roles are similar or different.

What is clear, is that the experiences of Pat, Kathy, Kito, and many other compassionate neighbours, resonate strongly with the notion of community provided by others. MacQueen et al. (2001) identify a common definition of community provided by a diverse range of communities in the US. Drawing on the views of nearly 100 people, they suggest a common definition of community as a group of people with diverse characteristics who are linked by social ties, share common perspectives, and engage in joint action in geographical locations or settings. Similarly, the compassionate neighbours programme draws together individuals who are diverse in terms of ethnicity, experience, education, and social background. Despite that, they create strong relationships; share an aspiration to improve the quality of life of individuals who are seriously ill, and those of their carers and who work together to enable that to happen across East London.

Concluding thoughts

The research done by Sallnow confirms a close relationship between the motivation and experience of the compassionate neighbours as volunteers, and their identity as members of a community. There is a strong story of the mutuality of benefit in the relationships they enjoy in this role, and that these relationships are multi faceted—encompassing those enjoyed with community members, other compassionate neighbours, and people they meet in the hospice. The benefit is that of personal and social transformation—arising from a growing sense of empowerment and agency—being confident of making a difference and of being increasingly connected as a member of a number of different communities. As a result of galvanizing volunteer activity with a strong community focus, we see the start of a social movement. The value of this is lies in its potential to facilitate change well beyond the relationships established between compassionate neighbours and community members—the kind of upstream transformation that is inherent to societal change necessary to transform human experiences such as dying and loss. Such change has been noted in other parts of the world, such as Kerala (see Chapter 12), resulting in sustainable, community led solutions that equip them with the skills and confidence to change not only experiences of death, dying, and loss but to tackle broader issues of social justice, cohesion, and compassion.

References

Baum, F. and Ziersch, A. (2003) Social capital. *Journal of Epidemiology and Community Health* **57**(5): 320–23.

Burbeck, R., Low, J., Sampson, E., Bravery, R., Hill, M., Morris, S., Ockenden, N., Payne, S., and Candy, B. (2014) Volunteers in specialist palliative care: A survey of adult services in the United Kingdom. *Journal of Palliative Medicine* **17**(5): 568–74.

Karapliagkou, A. and Kellehear, A. (2014) *Public health approaches to end of life care: a toolkit.* Public Health England and National Council for Palliative Care. Available from: http://www.ncpc.org.uk/sites/default/files/Public_Health_Approaches_To_End_of_Life_Care_Toolkit_WEB.pdf

Kellehear, A. (2005) *Compassionate Cities.* London: Routledge.

MacQueen, K.M., McLellan, E., and Trotter, R.T. (2001) What is community? An evidence-based definition for participatory public health. *Am J Public Health* **91**(12): 1929–38.

National Institute for Health and Care Excellence. (2014) *Community engagement to improve health. NICE local government briefings, 2014.* Available from: http://publications.nice.org

O'Mara-Eves, A., Brunton, G., McDaid, D., et al. (2013) Community engagement to reduce inequalites in health: a systematic review, meta-analysis and economic analysis. *Public Health Res* **1**(4): 1–548.

Richardson, H. (2012) A public health approach to palliative care in East London: wearly developments, challenges and plans for the future. In: Sallnow, L., Kumar, S. and Kellehear, A. (eds) *International perspectives on public health and palliative care.* Abingdon: Routledge, (pp. 110–22).

Sallnow, L., Kumar, S., and Kellehear, A. (eds) (2012) International Perspectives on Public Health and Palliative Care. Abingdon: Routledge.

Sallnow, L., Richardson, H., Murray, S.A., and Kellehear, A. (2017) Understanding the impact of a new public health approach to end of life care: a qualitative study of a community led intervention. *Lancet* (23 February 2017) doi: http://dx.doi.org/10.1016/S0140-6736(17)30484-1.

Scott, R. (2015) We cannot do it without you—the impact of volunteers in UK hospices. *European Journal of Palliative Care* **22**(2): 80–3.

South, J. (2014) *A guide to community-centred approaches for health and wellbeing* (full report). London: Public Health England.

Szreter, S. and Woolcock (2004) Health by association? Social capital, social theory and the political economy of public health. *International Journal of Epidemiology* **33**(4): 650–67

Wegleitner, K., Heimerl. K., and Kellehear, A. (2015) *Compassionate Communities: Case Studies from Britain and Europe.* Abingdon: Routledge.

Chapter 15

In our own words ...

Ros Scott

Introduction

I would first to acknowledge the contributions from Rosalma Badino, Italy: Heidi Hodder and Donna MacKenzie, Australia; Irina Padureanu, Romania; Sainudeen Muhammed, India; Miriam Bowers, the United States of America (USA); Kim Martin, Scotland United Kingdom (UK) Agnieszka Kaluga, Poland, and to thank them for their willingness and openess in sharing their personal stories.

Terry Pratchett once suggested that 'people merely become part of other's narratives if they don't tell their own story' (Pratchett, 2011). Much is written about volunteering, often by paid staff or researchers, rather than by the volunteers themselves. For too long volunteers in hospice and palliative care have been part of someone else's story.

From papers and articles we know about volunteer motivations, the roles they undertake, their value, and how they are managed. But how much do we know about their experiences of being a volunteer? What happens in that unique space that volunteers inhabit—between patient, family, and the multi-professional team? What does it mean to the volunteer?

Telling stories is one of the earliest and most common forms of communication throughout the world. History and culture are often passed down through the generations by the telling of stories. Cooper et al. (1994) describe stories as a 'gift' (p. 1). Recounting stories in a palliative care context may help the storyteller to share all types of experiences, some difficult; reflect and make sense of these, offering opportunities for personal insights, and enabling growth.

This chapter has tried to capture the voices of volunteers from Italy, Australia, Romania, India, the USA, UK and Poland who have generously offered to share their stories with us in their own words. Volunteers were invited to share their experiences and were given three broad questions to prompt their thinking: 'What do you do as a volunteer?', 'What does it mean to you?' and 'What more would you like to do?'.

The stories are both moving and compelling in their openness of very personal and individual experiences.

Story 1

Rosalma Badino, volunteer, Gigi Ghirotti Hospice, Genoa, Italy

'I am an Italian volunteer working at Gigi Ghirotti Hospice in Genoa. To be able to be really helpful, I try to bring myself to this experience, after having explored my personal suffering. I would like to share my experience of working with a lady that I met some months ago.

She was 80 years old, arrived at the Hospice in the morning and I met her during my afternoon shift. She was very angry with everybody, she felt as if all people round her (nurses, and other staff) laughed at her and made fun of her. Her words were confused: she was seeing things that were not there. She was really upset and did not accept any reasoning. Caring for her was exhausting.

I entered the room realizing that the situation was difficult to face. The patient looked very distressed, in a trance-like state, struggling with visions of things that were not there. I sat quietly by the bedside, listening to her complaints, nodding sometimes, showing understanding and sympathy and trying to create an intimacy as in a friendship. I tried to help to reassure her about what she believed that she was seeing. She looked at me, hopefully I was able to reassure her. She relaxed.

Then she turned her head to one side and talked quietly with her husband who had died previously. She was aware that he had died the year before, but believed that he had now been allowed to visit her . . . She was disappointed: 'why he does not answer me?' 'Maybe he is thinking . . . he will answer you later . . .' I said. The lady settled and slowly fell asleep. She died a few hours later. After this experience I learned not to be afraid to be with patients in their own world and beliefs.

I remember another patient who complained that she was very scared during the night; she did not know why. 'Stay here with me tonight, stay here please . . .' she pleaded, holding tightly my hand. Trying to soothe her, I talked about my own death: 'I don't know when it will come, when I will meet death. Then she relaxed and told quietly about her son and had a little dinner later. I had found a meeting point with her. Sometimes the effort to protect ourselves can create a barrier, a separation between the volunteer and the patient.

We don't have to be afraid to face our helplessness, but just bring to the bedside our passion and our fear, also. Patients will feel that we are participating in their inner suffering, and then they will feel better.

It is my opinion that we need to spend time reflecting to find the necessary peace of mind, inspecting our thoughts and feelings. Introspection has a strong potential to promote empathy and a very powerful energy. Those who decide to become volunteers with dying patients and want to be really helpful, must work on themselves, explore their personal suffering to get in touch with another human being without fear.

In our hospice we have great opportunities for personal development. One of these is to attend periodic meeting for discussions led by a psychologist where volunteers can meditate, share their experiences and improve their motivation.

I offer my presence and support to the patient as well as to relatives and friends, who often are anxious or overwhelmed when caring for a dying loved one. Being a calm presence, sitting together, talking and listening, sharing silence, listening to music, can be really helpful to them.

I consider it a privilege to be with dying people. I have learned to stay close to people I meet in every day life, with more understanding and empathy. I have learned to think not only that a person I met in the morning, maybe I will not meet in the evening again … but also that our life is so short and uncertain.'

Nagarjuna, a buddist philosopher, said: 'one dwells amid factors that can cause death just as a lamp that sits in gusting winds' (Nagarjuna n.d.).

Story 2

Heidi Hodder, volunteer, Sydney Local Health District Palliative Care Service, New South Wales, Australia

'I volunteer in palliative care in the community. This involves visiting my client once a week. Usually I take her to the hospital where she has massage therapy and physiotherapy, but sometimes we stay in her home and I give her a foot massage while we talk and her husband is able to go out and do some shopping.

My client is unable to walk and she feels very frustrated and upset about her physical condition. Before she became unwell she was the one taking care of her home and her family as well as working outside the home, it's very hard for her to adjust to being the one taken care of and there is a lot more conflict within the home since she lost her mobility due to a tumour. I think when we first met she wasn't sure what I could do for her other than transport but so often now she says to me "I'm so so lucky to have you." We talk about our families, cry together, hug each other. This role means a lot to me as I feel I'm making a positive difference to someone who is going through a really challenging time. My client talks a lot about her disappointment at having a terminal illness and losing her mobility, she expected to live well into old age like her mother and grandmother. She talks about her life regrets, happy memories, present ailments and worries. She cries and smiles a lot when we are together and I know it means a lot to her that I care and understand. We are from very different cultural backgrounds but definitely on the same wavelength.

There are lots of other things I would like to do as a volunteer but am not permitted to by regulations/staff attitudes. For example I would like to be able to take my client somewhere nice like a park by the water, or to a café or shopping. She has said many times how much she would like this but we have been told no when seeking permission. I understand that the staff want to protect my safety and time and I appreciate this but it would be good if the program were more flexible.'

Story 3

Irina Padureanu, Red Cross volunteer, Center of Palliative Care, Saint Nectarie, Romania

'I can't imagine life without the power of offering. I couldn't conceive such great beauty until I met Mrs. M. Her sparkling eyes were looking at us piercingly, she was smiling at us and with a calming voice she said "You are God's children, little girls and little boys". Frail hands were slowly rising from the bed of the hospital Saint Nectarie, a bed that was representing an end to a human's life, and she was squeezing my hand. I talked to her. I found out that she was living in (name of place), that she was alone for her entire life and that she never missed the opportunity to accommodate faithful travellers at her house. She was a wonderful woman, a woman who was holding me tight with her hands filled by a terrible illness and she was reciting a poem.

She was a pure soul who died not long after the New Year's Eve. I felt a strong sadness when I found out that both her body and soul had gone forever from this world. Mrs. M is one of many people I know who took their last breath to the Center of Palliative Care Saint Nectarie.

I started volunteering at the Red Cross, and every week I go there with my friends to talk to the patients, to give and receive smiles. But behind their smiles, is the sadness of taking their last walk to the hospital's bed. Sad faces of people who know that they'll leave behind a whole family. People who won't stop hoping that they will get better, that they will get out of the bed and run free to their own houses where family waits for them with their arms wide open. However, patients from this hospital ward will not get to go home. It was extremely sad but I understood that I'm not going there for myself. I'm going there because everyone deserves to leave this world reconciled with themselves. It is my way to offer something that can't be compared with an object or with a 'thank you', it is my way to offer love and hope.

Days are passing by, people are coming and going, but we stay here eternally anchored by the strong bond of love and smiles incessantly offered by people. It is an experience I will never forget. Thanks to volunteering at Red Cross

I learned what means to cherish everything I have, I learned to have hope and to love! Thank you!'

Story 4

Sainudeen Muhammed, volunteer, India

'My name is Sainudeen Muhammed, and for me volunteering is not something for which an extra effort is to be made. It is part of my day to day life. This "streak" runs in me from my early days. As a young boy I used to do odd jobs to earn pocket money and always used to share a part of that with people I thought needed support. Later when I lived, struggled and worked in many cities in India, I closely watched the lives of marginalised people in the big cities and where ever possible continued to support such people.

My formal introductions to palliative care happened in the mid nineties through some common friends who were part of the Pain & Palliative Care Society (which pioneered the community based palliative care programmes) at Kozhikode. Then I joined the rehabilitation initiatives of the organisation and travelled extensively in North Kerala to visit patients and families trying to understand their lives and to see what kind of support will suit them the best. This was a great experience.

Many carers have to take a day off to take their ailing family member to palliative care centre or to report to collect medicines. This affected them financially and friends and I thought that an evening out-patient clinic would solve the issue to some extent. The clinic started in 2003 which was later, in 2006, converted in to a fully fledged home care programme in line with the evolving community owned palliative care network in Kerala and care is taken to patients' home. A new organisation, Palliative Care Society, was formed to take local lead in enrolling community volunteers and raising resources. I took up the task of leading the organisation. In the last ten years I have worked as CEO and chairman of the organisation. In addition to visiting patients at home, I oversee the administration, home care services, fundraising and HR management. My main achievements during this period apart from steering the programme through the early forming period are:

1. Creating a decentralised network for palliative care where more and more local people will involve in the activities leading to better coverage and resource mobilisation to ensure the sustainability of the programme.

2. Collaborating with the Institute of Palliative Medicine, Kozhikode to start a 24 hour home care (first in the country) where palliative care patients and their families from the city area can request for emergency home care services even in the middle of the night.

The organisation now has eight home care teams going out every day. They take care of around 1,200 patients at any given point of time and have a support base of 300 active volunteers in the city. Creating an infrastructure for this would not have happened without the community taking ownership of the programme. While I did all these things as a volunteer I was also running a successful courier business in the region.

I want to bring in more volunteers into the network. The only way to sustain the community owned programmes is to invest in people. They will help to identify the needy, assess the local needs in a better way, find resource from the neighbourhood and act as quality control to the service. Our collective aspiration is to create a network of services in the city which will be able to see a patient with in twenty minutes of calling the home care service.

This voluntary work means a lot to me. I am fulfilling my responsibility towards the society where there are inequalities due to various reasons. Chronic illness is one of them. This is a way to give back to the society and most satisfying part is that one can see, right in front of his/her eyes, how their help makes a difference to peoples' lives. This completes my life.'

Story 5

Miriam Bowers, volunteer, Hospice of the Bay, San Francisco, California, USA

'As part of the hospice team, I have done whatever I could to help. There were no limitations to what I was willing to do. I am trained as a Patient Care Volunteer. In this role I serve both patients and families.

As a volunteer I found that one quickly gains experience and confidence in assessing the situation on arrival, and in filling the needs that arise, graciously, and as best I could. With gentle inquiry or through quiet observation, I would ascertain:

- Does the family need kind words, companionship or just conversation?
- Or does the patient want me to read aloud from a book or magazine?
- Or does the patient prefer a quiet presence? In time I understood that not every moment of silence needed to be filled with talk. Just being there was enough. In some cases they wanted no company at all and I was content to sit in another room.

In my early days of volunteering, almost three decades ago, I often did household chores such as cooking, light cleaning and even gardening; and sometimes I walked the family dog or took the patient for a ride in the country or to the local grocery store. With regard to practical care, I transferred patients from their bed to a chair and back, took patients to the toilet, sometimes while tethered by a long tube to an oxygen tank.

But times change, along with regulations, equipment and improved supplies. Now-a-days I usually read to a patient or sit near the bedside, available but reflective, and sometimes engaged in my own activity. The rustle of paper or the motions of hand-sewing is somehow soothing to them. Plus, some families will say that they feel less guilty about the unpaid, volunteer hours when they see that I have brought a personal project to work on.

I began as a hospice volunteer in my mid-40s. Some of my friends would inquire: 'Isn't being a volunteer depressing?' Without hesitation I would reply: 'No, it's not.' What has been far more difficult to explain to them is why the experience brings me back, again and again, week after week, year after year for nearly 30 years.

While my time spent with those I serve is measurable, the returns from it are not. How does one put into words the peace, the stillness, and the state of grace that envelops a person who has surrendered wholly to their life-limiting circumstance?

Over these many years I feel patients somehow know they are not their body; they seem to know there is something beyond this life. For me this is still a concept with which I struggle and so it is a great privilege to witness their true detachment.

Incapacity, loss and sorrow are superseded by poise, acceptance and a lightness that fills the space. The value of that is incalculable. Without a doubt, being a volunteer has been one of the most meaningful experiences of my 75 years of life.

What I miss most is permission to feed a patient. I understand the liability involved, but the prohibition has made it more difficult to serve some families. For example one family I served took a break each week from caring for their elderly mother and went to a restaurant for dinner. It would have been more convenient for them had I been able to assist the 90-some year old woman with her meal by feeding her. As it was, I could only heat the meal.'

Story 6

Kim Martin, volunteer, Rachel House Children's Hospice, Kinross, Scotland, UK

'I volunteer twice a week for Children's Hospices Across Scotland at Rachel House Children's Hospice. As a care support volunteer, I help the care team with a variety of tasks. These vary from helping with the children's personal care, washing and dressing etc. and spending time with siblings; this can be simply playing with the children, reading stories or taking part in activities, housekeeping tasks like stripping the beds when the children are going home. This is a relatively new role and it has been nice getting to work with lots of different members of staff and getting to know them, the children and families better.

I volunteer because I think it's important to give something back to the community, and I can't think of anything more rewarding to do in my spare time than come to Rachel House. Volunteering here also gives me the opportunity to refresh and strengthen my previous support work skills, with the added bonus of working with a really supportive, great bunch of people. It's a difficult job to do day in and day out, and I think the atmosphere here at Rachel house is that of a family, with every area working together and supporting each other in order to provide the best level of care. I feel really honoured to have been given the opportunity to be a small part of that, and to be able to work alongside people that have an amazing wealth of knowledge.

Moving forward I think I would really like to be given the opportunity to complete some more training, mainly because I would like to be able to do more to help and support the care team. For me personally, volunteering here is not simply about me giving my time, it's about me being given the opportunity to be constantly learning and, developing skills and knowledge. I feel that by being able to attend some in-house training courses, would allow for me to be able to give more back to Rachel House. It may sound to be a cliche but, my experience of volunteering is, that whatever I give to the role I'm rewarded tenfold, and if I could do it more often I would!

To me being a volunteer in a children's hospice means being able to help take a little bit of the weight off the staff, so they can focus on the most important tasks. It means for a little while being able to help families who are going through challenging times. It also means feeling honoured to be allowed in, by the families during these times and of course sharing happy moments too, of which there are many in Rachel House.

I've learned that no matter how inconsequential something may seem to the outside world it can mean so much more in Rachel House, asking a family member if they would like a cup of tea, what they have planned for the day and what kind of a night's sleep did they have, means a lot to those who very rarely have time to focus on themselves. I've learned that one of the best things to do on a Thursday morning is getting beaten at table football by two siblings! I've also learned, that a little smile, a blink of an eye, a chuckle of laughter and a thumbs up, can mean more than a thousand spoken words.'

Story 7

Agnieszka Kaluga, volunteer, Palium Hospice, Poznań, Poland

'Above all as a volunteer I am by the patients' side and I give them time. Mostly I listen, engage in conversation, laugh with them, sometimes I hold them by their hand and I read. I help with mealtimes, I take them on walks and if the patient needs something, I will go shopping for them. We look at family photos together, we watch films, news on the TV, and we listen to music. Sometimes I am a companion for patients when they are being transferred by ambulance to another hospital for tests. I talk with their family members—I try to support and relieve these people by persuading them to go home to relax, and by offering to take over some tasks while they are organising and taking care of their own lives/chores outside of the hospice. I assist in patient care, changing bed sheets, tidying cupboards, making tea and coffee, moisturising patients' lips and their skin, I cut patients finger and toe nails, and if necessary I change their incontinence pads.

As I have several years experience as a volunteer, I introduce new volunteer candidates to the ward, I show them how to be a companion to patients and how to manage and cope with their own emotions. At times, I lead lectures and training (for both medical and nursing students). I am also involved in various external activities (volunteer initiatives) for the benefit of the hospice. Sometimes I write notes on the hospice web page, I assist in the editing of a range of letters including thank-you notes and invitations.

Additionally I attend the funerals of my patients, I also make home visits to their families. I once invited a young widow and her three children to my home for Christmas, however these types of situations are infrequent. When I visit a patient at home, I help in the preparation of dinner, doing shopping and laundry. I help in the organisation of charity concerts for the hospice, sometimes I give interviews, I hand out brochures/pamphlets to my friends that promote the support of my hospice, I lead classes in high schools and I show young people what a volunteer is and does and how everyone can join in and contribute to services in the hospice.

Being a volunteer is a luxury, as it means that I can give and I have a way to give. This is a great freedom, as I decide how much and when I can help. This liberty also gives me the ability to say no to nurses if they suggest that I take on some of their professional duties. In the hospice, I am there for the patients, not for the nurses/medical staff. I do not go there to do the work of someone else, I go there so that patients feel cared for, valued and respected. My priority is always the patient and their family, as these are the people that I become close to and it is their requests that I am inclined to fulfill.

Being a volunteer is a journey to self-development and at the same time. It is a product of your own development, as you are ready to get out of your comfort zone and your own environment and meet others—those who have less (time, health, money, presence, closeness, love) and need support. One effect of volunteer work was my decision to attain a second degree in psychology. This was a big challenge for me, to start university again at the age of 35. I succeeded, and

I know that I was only brave enough to embark on that journey thanks to my role as a volunteer.

Being a volunteer is an obligation and a responsibility, you cannot engage in a relationship with a patient and then leave them. Being a hospice volunteer changes you—it taught me to keep my opinions to myself, I definitely do not hand out advice as readily as I used to, I listen more. Volunteer work is a school of tolerance. I meet many different people (world views, education, religion) and I know how to respect them all. Being on the ward in the role of a volunteer is an important part of my life, and I do not intend to let it go.'

Reflections and conclusion

The aim of this chapter was to open a window into volunteering lives and to understand more clearly what it is really like to be a volunteer supporting those facing the end of life.

These stories so willingly shared have painted a rich picture of volunteering in different countries, settings and experiences; of sensitivity and intuitiveness. The stories describe a unique role of human interaction borne out of a desire to walk alongside another person as they face the end of life. They tell of the challenges faced in being within this space and of the significant rewards that such volunteering can bring.

It seems fitting, therefore that the last words in this chapter should be from a volunteer:

Thoughts on being a palliative volunteer

It's the first knock on the door that's hardest,
the not knowing.
not knowing what they are expecting,
these people near the brink of death –
mostly couples –
one to die, one to be left behind.
that first knock: what will they see?
what will they read in my face
that will let me into their lives
for this brief time
near the end of their ordeal?
maybe they see negatives first:
no threat, no fear, no agenda on my part,
then, hopefully, the positives of the job description
which could read something like:
'no formal training required
but desirable qualities include:
a mind as broad as our brown land,
good timing,

sensitivity to others' needs and feelings,
no personal agenda, except to have none,
yet a wish to be there for them,
a gentle sense of humour,
enough personal integrity so as not to be
felled by the death blow when it comes,
availability,
flexibility,
and maybe some invisible, indispensable
personal salvations like
courage
commitment
and fortitude, whatever that is.
what sort of job is it
where not doing too much is most of the job?
we sit, we chat, we might
do a bit of shopping, a bit of cleaning,
cook a meal
offer a shoulder, or pass the tissues.
but mostly what we offer is intangible, more our presence
and in being present in our
witnessing of their passage
through this signal event in their lives.
there's the nub of it for me:
something about being invited
to witness
this mightiest of struggles.
what rare privilege this is.

Donna McKenzie, A Palliative Care Volunteer with the Nepean Hawkesbury Palliative Care Volunteer Service, Penrith, New South Wales, Australia. Reproduced courtesy of the author.

References

Cooper, P., Collins, R., and Saxby, H.M. (1994) *The power of story*. Melbourne: Macmillan Education Australia PTY Ltd.

Nagarjuna (n.d.). *A Buddhist Library, Contemplating the uncertainty of the time of death.* Available from: http://www.abuddhistlibrary.com/Buddhism/A%20-%20Tibetan%20Buddhism/Authors/Pabonkha%20Rinpoche/From%20'Liberation%20In%20Our%20Hands'-%20Impermance/VII/Contemplating%20the%20uncertainty%20of%20the%20time%20of%20death.htm

Pratchett, T. (2011) *The Amazing Maurice and His Educated Rodents*. London: Random House Children's Books, p. 148.

Chapter 16

Pulling it all together

Steven Howlett and Ros Scott

Introduction

In approaching this book we set out to gather accounts from different countries of the changing landscape of volunteering in hospice and palliative care. We sought to understand volunteering within the changing contexts of both palliative care and of volunteering. The book, therefore, explores volunteering through a number of lenses: the history and development of volunteering, the impact of political and legislative influences, approaches to management and training, how and why volunteering is changing and what makes it successful. Authors have also described the challenges of supporting and managing volunteers through change. Others describe community models of volunteering, whether initiated by organizations, or by the community itself and the challenges experienced in providing palliative care in countries where the demand is overwhelming and resources scarce. Most powerful of all was hearing from volunteers themselves, how they experience what they do, and what it means to them to volunteer in this field.

It is hard to do justice to the richness, diversity, and complexity of volunteering as described by the authors in a summary chapter. The aim of this final chapter, therefore, is to give a brief overview of a few of the editors' impressions, ending with some thoughts on what lies ahead for volunteering in this sector.

Volunteering and the development of hospice and palliative care

Each country profiled in this book started from a similar realization that people at the end of life needed care and that families and carers also needed help and support at this time. And yet care, other than that by families, was often missing, and death was something not to be talked of. Each of our authors trace how this began to change. But it is interesting to see the diverse ways in which volunteering in hospice and palliative care emerged in each country; from volunteer-led non-medical movements, to physician-led services, whether promoted or opposed by political movements or religious groups. For example, in Austria (Chapter 4), and Poland (Chapter 7), religious groups were influential in the development of services. By contrast in Germany (Chapter 6), churches opposed the development of the hospice movement through misguided assumptions of links to the holocaust and euthanasia. Despite the different drivers for providing care, the work of Dame Cicely Saunders figures highly. Recognized as the founder of the modern hospice movement in the UK, and St Christopher's hospice in London, her influence in a number of other countries is plain to see. But even though her legacy is obvious, there are different interpretations of how to implement care delivery. Some countries went on to develop similar types of hospice care organizations such as in Poland (Chapter 7), Canada (Chapter 8), whilst in others, such as the Netherlands (Chapter 5), locating care through a hospice building was thought to be 'too institutionalized'. What is interesting is that despite the different approaches, and even in countries where medical professionals initiated palliative care, a groundswell of volunteering activity sprang up in response to local needs. The involvement of volunteers is the common factor across all the chapters and each makes clear that volunteering is vital to the future of hospice and palliative care.

Our authors have volunteers at the centre of their accounts and the chapters show how volunteers both influence, and are influenced by cultural, historical, and political traditions and have played a key role in the initiation and ongoing development of services. What authors describe as they give us the history of hospice and palliative care in their country, are the results of how these factors mix and unfold. The vision of Cicely Saunders for volunteering is noticeable in many accounts. Even where, as in the Netherlands, there was not a replication of hospice care as in St Christopher's hospice in London, her determination that people at the end of life should be cared for and supported was underpinned by a belief that volunteers had a part to play. Very importantly, her idea that those volunteers should both represent and reach out into the community does seem to be a universal aim of services. This aspect of hospice and palliative care still echoes through many of the care systems reported.

That history gives us a landscape, or canvas, over which new approaches are laid. But of course, as each new challenge, issue, or approach lands on existing infrastructure so it interacts in different ways. It was through setting the scene in the first two chapters that we hoped to show the context for the changes identified within each chapter.

Changing motivations

We noted in Chapter 1 that motivations have been extensively researched. The models that research give us to work with are useful in that as we read each of the chapters we get the impression that volunteer motivations appear to be very similar regardless of culture or setting. Sallnow (Chapter 12) recounts how volunteers in a neighbourhood scheme in the UK talk of having a chance to exercise compassion and deepen feelings of community belonging, themes echoed in the volunteer stories in Chapter 15. Kiyange (Chapter 11), provides an excellent overview of palliative care across many African countries and noted that themes of compassion were strong here too with palliative care volunteering built out of cultural traditions of community care. Yet, Kiyange's chapter also provides an illustration of motivations driven by a desire to attain paid employment at the same time as being an expression of these traditional cultural values of community help and care. Already with just these two examples we can see that altruism exists alongside more evident instrumental motivations in that volunteers are driven by desires to give freely of themselves to others, but also that volunteering can be of direct benefit to the volunteer. As we noted in Chapter 1, research into motivations describe a shifting balance between these 'giving and receiving' motivations and organizations are changing how they involve volunteers to provide a meaningful experience for the volunteer. That could mean helping the volunteer to feel that they are giving back to the community or providing an experience which will enable them to gain the experience and skills applicable to other areas of their lives.

Historically, it seems in many countries' volunteers in this field were driven primarily by altruistic reasons. Whilst this still shows as a strong theme in India (Chapter 12), and for some volunteers in other countries, it would appear that this is gradually changing. It seems that all the academics and practitioners writing in this book highlight that time is a key constraint for volunteers today. Some solutions offered by authors in addressing volunteer time constraints include dividing work into more time-limited opportunities; this is a trend echoed in volunteering in general. Volunteers, therefore, with less time to give, seek personal and professional development and as a result expect more meaningful and responsible roles. The implication is that organizations (and their managers) will need to work harder to provide that experience.

Will how organizations approach managing the commitment asked of potential volunteers be a key indicator of successful recruitment and retention? Certainly recognizing time constraints is necessary, but however much time a volunteer gives, it needs to be time well spent and to match both their expectations and the needs of the organization.

Even when we acknowledge that motivations need to be understood as both altruistic and instrumental, and that there is a general trend towards volunteers offering less time (see Chapter 1), we also must recognize the need to understand specific contexts. For example, the Africa chapter (Chapter 11), highlights the value of a stipend in attracting volunteers, and yet we need to understand that this is born from the paucity of employment opportunities in poor areas and the poverty of the volunteers themselves, it is not necessarily an indication that all volunteer programmes need to consider payments. Meanwhile volunteers' desire to acquire skills is something highlighted in all chapters. At the same time, the influence of culture and tradition is strong. The underlying story from our chapters is that *something* needs to be offered over and above, or as well as, an opportunity to reward our altruistic motivations. In Africa it may be a stipend. In other countries it is noticeable that volunteering in hospice and palliative care offers the chance to acquire a sophisticated set of skills. For example, countries such as Austria and Germany (Chapters 4 and 6) among others, provide a very structured education programme with skills that could transfer to many other aspects of a volunteer's life (and career choices). Could it be argued that the need to fulfil the requirements of training programmes restricts who can or will volunteer? Maybe these models, for all their strengths, would not work for volunteers with limited time who just want to give a few hours, who want to 'lend a hand'. On the other hand, palliative care can be demanding, patient and family needs may be complex, and volunteers need to be effectively prepared to cope with the varying demands that will be made of them. Interestingly, however, drawing on the volunteer stories, what comes through is as much about how volunteers feel about themselves and what they do, as it is about any tangible training and qualifications. That is to say, while managers worry about motivations, skills, and training, volunteers tell stories of human experiences and meaning.

In the end the chapters in this book will not provide answers as to what motivates the modern volunteer. Instead, taken collectively, they emphasize what a volunteer manager, or palliative care programme developer, or indeed a policy-maker needs to consider. The underlying factor is that volunteers need a purpose and this can be variously interpreted. It can be that a motivation is satisfied or it could be that volunteering contributes to an understanding of the self and others. The difference is how that works in practice. For Sallnow (Chapter 12), the neighbourhood project used 'neighbour' as a deliberate word. It allowed for a less constrained role where the families helped to define the help needed. What it does is free the volunteer to define their own identity as volunteer/neighbour/helper. In the Netherlands (Chapter 5), the complexity is captured in the exploration of the concept of 'being there'. Volunteers are interviewed and, if suitable, go on to attend seven training sessions. The training itself (as in a number of other countries) acts as a selection process and volunteers can decide after training that volunteering may not be what they want to do. Those that do go on engage with 'being there' as Chapter 5 describes. However, as that chapter notes that while the concept of 'being there' forms a strong part of a volunteers identity, it is not so easy to define. The chapter asks: 'Can it be considered a competence? A talent? A skill? Can it be learned and improved? Is selection possible based on performed quality of being there?'

Indeed, the complexity does not stop there. If we want to learn from the idea of expressing volunteer purpose in terms of 'being there' we should consider how it is affected by culture. Anecdotal evidence suggests that some patients and families may find it easier to accept practical help rather than admit that they need emotional support, interpreted by some as weakness or failure. Yet the connection with the volunteer often grows into something deeper, the volunteer's role in the fullest sense of 'being there' gradually develops. In other words, in such a context, what starts as volunteering being defined in quite task-oriented terms, may develop into something that is more explicable in terms of what it means to volunteer.

Such are the complexities of organizing volunteering in a sensitive area such as palliative and end-of-life care, across a range of formal and more informal organizations, against a back drop of changing motivations, and increasing demand. Is it any wonder that managing volunteers has become more complicated? We return to this below when we reflect on how volunteer management compares across countries.

Organizing and empowering volunteering

The challenges facing palliative care services around the world are highly significant as outlined by Payne and Morris in Chapter 2. Indeed, this is a recurring theme throughout most chapters. Authors reinforce the scale of these challenges, whether as a result of aging populations resulting in a significant demand for palliative care, the increasing complexity of palliative care patient needs, sheer population size as in India (Chapter 12), or the significant burden arising from the scale of communicable diseases in Africa (Chapter 11).

This in turn has a significant impact on volunteering. There is universal agreement that volunteers are vital to hospice and palliative care, now and in the future. As we have seen from the preceding chapters, volunteers under-take a wide range of roles and activities, ranging from the governance and leadership of some services, delivering elements of care, providing psychosocial support to patients and families, offering respite for family carers through practical support with everyday tasks, and supporting services with administration and fundraising. Each role and each volunteer plays an important part in contributing to the whole within these services. However, as we have heard from some authors, sometimes the diversity and value of this is not always recognized. This in itself poses challenges for the organization of volunteering.

Indeed, there is also consensus that increasing volunteer involvement is essential in enabling services to respond to the changing palliative care landscape and the rapidly growing demand around the world. Might this see a need for new and innovative volunteer roles or changes to training to empower volunteers to work alongside a population with increasingly complex needs? This, at a time when the nature of volunteering itself is shifting. We have noted motivations are changing, however, there are other challenges facing volunteer-involving organizations, including how we conceptualize and describe volunteering, approaches to management, and the availability of current and prospective volunteers.

There is more to volunteering than purely meeting need, however, and it is suggested in Chapter 2 that volunteer involvement enables creativity through helping multi-disciplinary teams to 'forge innovative alliances to shape the compassionate care of people facing the final stages of life'. However, in many of the chapters, volunteering is also about 'becoming who the other person needs' (Chapter 5), regardless of how the introduction and relationship begins. Authors in this book have shown that volunteering is so much more than an inventory of different services. Perhaps, by attempting to define what volunteering is and is not, we limit the benefits that volunteers can bring to patients and their families.

The challenge highlighted in this collection seems to be the drive towards more management which answers one set of organizational needs but could have the unintended consequence of making it more difficult to let the ideals of volunteering flourish. We were struck by Hartley's chapter (Chapter 13) whereby the evident need to manage change raised so many challenges. The need to adapt to survive in a changing environment as Hartley describes makes complete sense. But we also noted that this led to thinking whereby managers felt the compulsion to keep volunteers close where they could 'keep an eye on them'. As we noted in Chapter 1, Rochester's analysis of the rise of the management model, predicts just such a response to management challenges. The need for management we do not think will change; but maybe if we are to develop volunteer management into a profession the importance of how to work simultaneously with quite different models of participation needs to be developed. Academics and researchers can help practitioners in this quest.

Perhaps a starting place (and maybe this is a modern twist on palliative care volunteering beyond hospice walls that Cicely Saunders argued for), is to consider the language we use and to start to think and talk more about partnership with communities and individuals, encouraging engagement at a level of one person reaching out to another. This is not saying that we advocate a move that merely relabels against management terms, or that careful selection, initial training, and supervision of volunteers is not required. Quite the reverse—it is about these being reflective, values-based processes that not only prepare volunteers to provide effective support, but empower them to use their own skills and experiences and to respond appropriately to the many different scenarios that they will meet. It involves using language that is inclusive and encourages all to think of volunteers as partners and co-creators. We think that will strengthen what it means to volunteer and help us avoid further drift into thinking about volunteering as paid work without pay. It calls for quite brave approaches to a management attitude that empowers volunteers as well as providing leadership.

The challenges noted in this book are those facing volunteering in general and in hospice and palliative care specifically. In Chapter 1, Howlett describes a relatively stable international picture with no obvious upward trend in the number of people who volunteer. Yet in Australia (Chapter 10), statistics suggest that fewer people are volunteering. In the UK recent studies suggest that volunteering are giving less time (Chapter 1) and this is echoed by authors in other countries. While this may be a trend in volunteering generally, it is noticeable, however, that there is less concern; that palliative care struggles to find volunteers. Scott (Chapter 3) makes the point that despite changes in volunteering in hospices and palliative care services in the UK, attracting volunteers is generally not problematic. On the one hand that is good for the continuation of services, perhaps we may argue that the 'steady state' of volunteering might lead to some complacency that we do not need to worry for the future. Yet the notion of being aware of changing motivations and expectations, new approaches to organizing and managing volunteers, not to mention the increasing complexity of patients' conditions, means that we cannot assume that we can approach volunteering in the future in the same way as we have in the past.

Authors describe the management challenges of organising and empowering volunteers. Some note the restricted role of volunteers as a direct result of the 'professionalization' of volunteering and of standardizing training and supervision (Chapter 6). Others have described the role of volunteers as 'shrinking' as a consequence of the complexity and requirements of hospice and palliative funding as in the USA (Chapter 9), where the role of volunteers is not explicit. How can we ensure that the importance of volunteering within organizations is recognized by policy-makers and that meeting regulatory requirements does not present barriers to volunteering? Volunteering is recognized by governments, but often in the tangible terms of making resources go further or helping people back into work. It is a challenge for volunteering in hospices and palliative care, but as previously mentioned in Chapter 2, the recently developed European Association for Palliative Care (EAPC) Charter on Volunteering in Hospice and Palliative Care attempts to address this and seeks to encourage individuals, and national and local organizations to consider and take action on some of these issues (see www.eapcnet.eu/Themes/Resources/VolunteeringCharter. aspx). Through this work the value of volunteering in hospice and palliative care is underlined and its importance as a key resource; more that 'money saved and skills learned' emphasized.

Whilst most authors identify fairly stable 'types' of volunteers in terms of age and gender, a younger volunteer profile is also emerging in a number of countries. For example, Paleri and Sallnow specifically note the younger age profile of volunteers within one neighbourhood scheme in India compared to those in other parts of the country (Chapter 12). It is also of note that in some children's services in the UK that a younger volunteering profile is more dominant. How can we ensure that we 'grow' the next generation of hospice and palliative care volunteers, not to mention staff, by encouraging young people to engage as volunteers?

Meeting the challenges

We have looked at what is happening to volunteering generally and compared research and trends to what is happening in volunteering in hospices and palliative care. But now we want to turn that around and look to see how volunteering in hospices and palliative care is moving forward to meet challenges.

As previously mentioned the EAPC Charter developed by the EAPC Task Force on Volunteering in Hospice and Palliative Care (EAPC Charter, 2017) argues that it is imperative to 'recognise volunteers as a third resource alongside professional care and family care, with its own position, identity and value'. Failing to accept this overlooks the vital role of volunteers, the psychosocial and practical support so essential to truly holistic care, not to mention the sustainability of services as highlighted by Scott in Chapter 3. Drawing out from our authors we see that taking this a step further Paleri and Sallnow (Chapter 12), give examples of projects led by communities where volunteers have leadership roles and where volunteers are in fact 'pillars rather that fillers' (page 215). Whilst this may be at odds with those hierarchical, management models in place in other countries, perhaps it is a concept that could change our constructs around the role of volunteers. Is it possible to begin to see volunteers as experts in their field rather than as 'assistants to experts' (Chapter 10)? This is an example of how we see a language developing that keeps the essence of volunteering as help freely given rather than a form of non-paid work. In fact we think this works across cultures. In resource-poor countries volunteering might be construed as 'non-paid work' because it is the only way that some services continue to exist, but in fact, as our chapters show, it is in these locations that more community involvement practices have developed. In other countries volunteering exists in a structured framework with highly developed volunteer management. In the UK, for example, Hartley emphasizes the need for management as organizations cope with a changing policy and practice environment. The authors in each chapter point to the successes of maintaining services and we draw from this the importance of volunteer management. But at the same time, we reflect on how the community model offers more empowerment for volunteers. We consider whether that may lead to volunteers constructing a meaning of their volunteering that is as important as the obvious gains of transferrable skills from the workplace model. At the very least, we wonder if this may not be a productive area for more research.

Findings from research from Age UK discussed by Payne and Morris in Chapter 2 suggest that volunteering could itself be seen as a specialist service. This is an interesting perspective and may be welcomed by those who have campaigned for better recognition of volunteering. This is already evident in the accounts from some of our authors and in others' ideas the groundwork is there. In a majority of countries volunteers are being trained to an extremely high standard. The question then comes back to the one we ask throughout—how that specialist service is led. Is there a tension between this approach and community engagement models or can an accommodation be reached? Can making volunteering a 'specialist service' still embraces the ethos and freedom that is volunteering?

What volunteers say about volunteering

Having considered volunteering from organizational and management perspectives, the implications of and for volunteering, it would be wrong to draw conclusions or to consider new approaches for the future without learning from the volunteers themselves. Their powerful and very personal accounts help our understanding of what it means to be a volunteer and inform our thinking about this vital partnership within hospice and palliative care.

Volunteers all tell of how important volunteering is to them; of the challenges faced, the journeys of self-development, and of being faced with their own mortality and that of others. Some speak of learning to let go of fear, accepting feelings of helplessness, and of the importance of reflecting upon and making sense of their own life experiences, hurts, and emotions.

Those who provide support to patients and families talk of the 'privilege' of such roles. Volunteers describe how much they value patients and families allowing them to share time and trusting them with confidences, emotions, and anxieties. They are open about sharing happy moments, along with experiencing their own sadness, whilst holding the sadness of others.

Whilst some volunteers spoke of the emotional and practical support that they gave, others gave examples of different activities. These included examples of leadership roles in developing new palliative care networks and projects; training and supporting new volunteers, in addition to raising awareness and raising funds. One volunteer expressed frustration at the limitations imposed on the volunteering role by regulations or by staff.

It would seem that for the volunteers in this book volunteering is very much part of life, giving new perspectives, insights, and confidence. They reflect on the value of giving to others, of developing patience and tolerance, and the rewards of making a real difference at a difficult time in peoples' lives. For many this gave them an appreciation of what is important in life and of how often actions can mean more than words.

Conclusion and reflections

All who contributed to this book all give a rich insight into the modern-day context of hospice and palliative care volunteering in different countries and settings. They illustrate just how much volunteering is shaped by history and culture. A rich and complex picture emerges of people reaching out to others in many ways and for many reasons. Volunteers shared the breadth and depth of their commitment and involvement, and the importance of individuals within the community reaching out to others. The authors leave us in no doubt that volunteers play an essential role in every aspect of hospice and palliative care and that their continued and increasing involvement will be essential in meeting the changing and increasingly complex demands of the future.

If they are to succeed in achieving this, however, managers, organizations, and policy makers must also take account of the changing context of volunteering within their culture and context. This offers many new and exciting opportunities to learn from each other; to explore new, innovative, and most importantly, culturally appropriate ways of working whilst engaging our communities and volunteers to inform the future.

For us this verse from the late Ivan Scheier, (Scheier, n.d.) one of the pioneers of thinking about volunteering, seems to sum up hospice and palliative care volunteering:

'Once, volunteering was for dreamers …
We were – and some still are – pioneers in compassionate enterprise.
It was the way we
Got good things done before there were big
Budgets or bureaucracies.
Once, volunteering was a legacy …
It was an inheritance from family, friends, or
Faith, an unself-conscious way of living out
Basic values.
Volunteer was just the way we were, a private matter of public consequence.
Once, volunteering was a power.
We didn't react to trends, we CAUSED them.
We didn't supplement staff, we CREATED them
Politicians didn't use us; we used them.
And we made dreams happen.
Once, volunteering was for dreamers.
May it soon be so again'

Ivan Scheier, Dreamcatcher-in-Residence, Voluntas
Reproduced with permission from *New Volunteerism Project:
The Ivan Scheier Archival Collection*, available online at
http://academic.regis.edu/volunteer/ivan/ from the Dayton
Memorial Library at Regis University, Denver, Colorado, USA.

References

EAPC *Charter on Volunteering* (2017). Accessed from: http://www.eapcnet.eu/Themes/Resources/VolunteeringCharter.aspx

Scheier, I (n.d.). Accessed from: http://academic.regis.edu/volunteer/ivan/sect05/sect05b.htm

Index

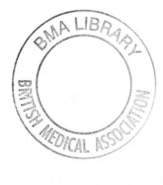